Advance Praise for *Dynamic DNA*

"Dr. Sharma's work has bridged the worlds of Ayurveda and modern science for three decades. In this new work, he makes the startling and insightful characterization that 'Ayurveda is epigenetics.' Contemporary evidence showing that genetic information from our life experience is carried across—and even changed within—generations is, he reveals, at the heart of what Ayurveda has described, and prescribed, for millennia.

By focusing on the inter-generational transfer of knowledge via the physics of DNA, Dr. Sharma makes the case for a physics of consciousness: of energy, its flow, and its essential nature as information. Some aspects of Vedic Science and its theory of energy are as yet untested by physics and medical science, and here Dr. Sharma and his coauthor, James G. Meade, PhD, build conceptual bridges that frame the direction for a new generation of insightful researchers. Dr. Meade brings his experience as a writer in the 'For Dummies' series, to work with Dr. Sharma in translating the challenging science of epigenetics and the multilayered concepts of Ayurveda into an accessible and fascinating reading experience."

—Gerard Bodeker, PhD
Dept. of Epidemiology, Columbia University, New York, USA
and Green Templeton College, University of Oxford, UK

"*Dynamic DNA* is not simply offering a fresh perspective on DNA, it is quietly offering nothing less than the solution to human suffering and, beyond even that, a vision of what comes when the pain is gone. The authors have unfolded the mysterious scientific subjects of DNA and kundalini. They have masterfully explained these topics with ample references from various scientific books and journals. They have used lucid language and given examples from day-to-day life.

Their deep insights in both the spiritual and scientific fields make the book an important reference on these subjects.

DNA was thought to be unchangeable. But scientific research has shown that DNA expression can be changed by epigenetics. The authors have explained in a simple way how the science of Ayurveda can affect DNA by turning genes on and off to change its expression. I recommend this book for every person who wants to know the secrets of DNA and Ayurveda."

—Prof. Emeritus Subhash Ranade
Chairman, International Academy of Ayurved
(www.ayurved-int.com)
Pune, India

"Connecting basic science, natural and integrative medicine with metaphysics, Dr. Sharma explains how the field of Ayurveda allows us to transform our lives by unfolding the full potential of our DNA. Epigenetics influences DNA expression through diet, behavior, meditation and environment. He takes us on a bold and thought-provoking journey toward understanding perfect health."

—Christopher Clark, MD
Coauthor, *Ayurvedic Healing*: *Contemporary
Maharishi Ayurveda Medicine and Science*
Founding medical director of the Raj Ayurvedic
Health Center and practicing psychiatrist

"One of the most important next steps in the evolution of modern medicine is understanding how our daily choices impact our DNA. Ayurveda is an ancient tool that allows us to address our modern health challenges through the deeper understanding of how we all control our genetic destiny. This book is a timely look into a subject that has the capacity to change the future of disease."

—Kulreet Chaudhary, MD
Neurologist and author of *The Prime:
Prepare and Repair Your Body for Spontaneous Weight Loss*

"Dr. Sharma is a conservative Western physician, yet his books are electrifying. *Freedom from Disease. The Answer to Cancer.* And now *Dynamic DNA* may be the biggest breakthrough of all. He goes deeper into the causes and treatments of disease than we ever have before, straight to the inner energy body and beyond. Wow."

—Suresh R. Chandra, MD

Emeritus Professor,
Department of Ophthalmology and Visual Sciences
University of Wisconsin Medical School, Madison, Wisconsin
Founder and Chairman, Combat Blindness International
www.combatblindness.org

"When we think mind/body, we tend to think of 'mind' as abstract. That is, we see the spiritual as wonderful but abstract. I love the way that Dr. Sharma here brings the spiritual into the everyday physical world, the world of DNA. If the spiritual is chemical, how many possibilities does that open? We can get our hands right on the spiritual. This is a book that opens new frontiers of understanding and, even better, of treatment."

—Nancy Liebler, PhD

Therapist and coauthor of *Healing Depression the Mind-Body Way: Creating Happiness with Meditation, Yoga, and Ayurveda*

"*Dynamic DNA* offers a new perspective looking at modern science through the ancient knowledge and wisdom of Ayurveda and Vedic Sciences. Dr. Sharma provides meaningful and thoughtful insights into the correlation between our diet, lifestyle choices, gene expression and evolution. In over 30 years of teaching and practicing Ayurveda worldwide, I believe this to be the most clearly articulated and illustrated reference on Ayurveda as epigenetics. Supported by extensive and groundbreaking research, yet accessible to all readers, this book is an indispensable resource for students, researchers, physicians, and all who seek to understand epigenetics leading us toward a conscious evolution of humanity."

—Prof. Shekhar Annambhotla, MD (Ayu)

President, AAPNA (Association of Ayurvedic Professionals
of North America, Inc., USA)
Ayurveda Director, International University of Yoga
and Ayurveda, Inc., USA

"Our knowledge of the genetic basis of life is rapidly expanding, and all the while we are becoming overwhelmed by an epidemic of chronic illness. Drs. Sharma and Meade achieve a synthesis of the ancient health science of Ayurveda with the most modern conclusions of epigenetics. In doing so, they uncover the key to health in our modern world. Their book plots a path back to nature along a modern freeway across an ancient landscape. A must-read for those in need of health, and who today doesn't need a way back to health?"

—Guy Hatchard, PhD
Natural health and Consciousness pioneer
Author of *Your DNA Diet*
New Zealand

"I bought 100 copies of Dr. Sharma's *The Answer to Cancer* to give to my patients. His collaboration with Dr. Meade creates a special chemistry—advanced scientific thinking presented in a compelling but understandable read. This latest undertaking, *Dynamic DNA*, presents new and useful knowledge about how to upgrade our DNA, the core of what makes us human. I appreciate the authors' insights and their sense of humor."

—John C. Peterson, MD

Dynamic
DNA

Dynamic DNA

Activating Your Inner Energy for Better Health

Hari Sharma, MD

and

James G. Meade, PhD

SelectBooks, Inc.
New York

This edition published by SelectBooks, Inc.
For information address SelectBooks, Inc., New York, New York.

First Edition

ISBN 978-1-59079-447-0

Library of Congress Cataloging-in-Publication Data
Names: Sharma, Hari, author.
Title: Dynamic DNA : activating your inner energy for better health / Hari
 Sharma, MD and James G. Meade, PhD.
Description: First edition. | New York : SelectBooks, [2018] | Includes
 bibliographical references and index.
Identifiers: LCCN 2017040814 | ISBN 9781590794470 (paperback book : alk.
 paper)
Subjects: LCSH: Medicine, Ayurvedic--Popular works. | Holistic
 medicine--Popular works.
Classification: LCC R605 .S4196 2018 | DDC 615.5/38--dc23 LC record
available at https://lccn.loc.gov/2017040814

Book design by Janice Benight

Manufactured in the United States of America
10 9 8 7 6 5 4 3 2 1

To modern medicine, for beginning to expose,
through genetics, the wonders of the universe inside

Acknowledgments

With sincere appreciation and gratitude, we want to thank Guru Dev (Swami Brahmananda Saraswati), Maharishi Mahesh Yogi, and other Vedic masters for their Vedic wisdom, including Swami Paramanand Giri Ji Maharaj, Paramahansa Yogananda, Swami Muktananda, and Swami Rama. We especially want to thank Maharishi for bringing out the Vedic knowledge in a very simplified and understandable way, making it available to anyone.

We also want to acknowledge our families for their patience and support during this ambitious undertaking.

Thanks to Nick Sharma and Ellen Kauffman for their beneficial editorial assistance. Thanks to Nina Meade for her support and organizing abilities. We also want to thank our publisher, SelectBooks and its head, Kenzi Sugihara, as well as Nancy Sugihara and Kenichi Sugihara, and our agent, Bill Gladstone of Waterside Productions, for all they have done.

Contents

Prologue:
Can Paradise Be Regained?

Life is frustrating. It seems we often take one step forward, two steps back. As the years accumulate, we grow in wisdom—which is fine. Meanwhile, as the years pass, our bodies lose more and more of their zip, our skin sags, and memory takes a somersault. We also accumulate baggage—broken relationships, job disappointments, missed opportunities to bring in "the big one," and a recurring sense of walking on a treadmill that seems to be taking us inexorably backward.

What would paradise regained look like? First of all, did we ever have it to lose? And if we did, we don't remember it. We're not even sure, truth be told, what paradise should be in the first place. The streets should be lined with gold. That, everyone agrees on. But then all the rest is up for debate. Will it be full of great food and exquisite relationships with only the best people? Is there wonderful TV there? Would it be a better place with or without cell phones? What would you do there?

The whole question of paradise and regaining it spins quickly out of control and into the ether. We don't know what it is. We don't know if we lost it. And we haven't a clue how to regain something when we're not even sure what it is.

Yet here in a science book we're looking at a material way to regain paradise and seeking it in a "chemical way" having to do with a substance in the body called DNA, an abbreviation for deoxyribonucleic acid, that we normally encounter only through watching crime dramas about DNA testing. We learned you can quickly identify a person by knowing his or her DNA (whatever that is).

And we suggest, too, that we don't have to know what paradise was or is. We just have to get the DNA working perfectly. In spite of all the stress of trudging through life and not really getting anywhere (with death guaranteed at the end), all we have to do is systematically purify the DNA. And then paradise awaits us. It doesn't matter what it is. We'll know it when we find it.

Working on the DNA sounds like something we can do, if we think of it as tinkering on a car or fixing up the house. We know about cleaning things up and getting them working right. We don't usually think of life as something we can treat that way. It's too relentlessly cruel and complicated. But the game changes when we think of just fixing something material.

What if we can lay out the elements of the body, lay out the characteristics of the energy world inside it and the pure consciousness within that, and just systematically work on them all? What if we forget ethics and metaphysics and just treat the whole package as something material?

And then, what if we fix what's wrong with it? What if we can change what's wrong through diet, lifestyle, stress management, and a healthy environment, supplemented with some powerful yogic techniques highlighted by meditation?

What if we can actually draw up the blueprint of regaining paradise? The poet John Milton tried, but he was limited to language to achieve his ends. We now have knowledge of DNA and of the one thing that opens the door to perfecting it—epigenetics. He had the words. But we can look at it all materially and say, you know, just maybe we can do it now. It is not the 1600s any more. It is the 21st century, and we are making breakthroughs with genetics every single day. Maybe the time has come for regaining paradise.

Note to the Reader

The contents of this book are not intended to diagnose, treat, cure, or prevent any disease. We are convinced that everyone should be aware of the knowledge and research reported in this book. That does not mean, however, that people who read this book should try to become medical experts on their own. Nothing in this book is meant to replace the advice of a physician. If you are sick, go to a doctor.

Part One

DNA:
The Cosmic Recorder

1

Sensitive DNA—
Our Link to the Universe

To begin to become acquainted with the deep levels of the body, we can start with the deepest level familiar to Western science because it is the deepest level we can see—the DNA. One of the best ways to get to know DNA is by observing how it behaves with disease.

Disease is when there is something wrong with the DNA. When you first think about DNA and disease, you may begin looking for hereditary diseases like hemophilia (of which Queen Victoria was a carrier). Look a little more closely, and cancer and heart disease begin to look hereditary. Widen the net, and what, if anything, gets left out? Is all disease hereditary? And if all disease is hereditary, what about all good things, like your wonderfully chiseled chin and your healthy skepticism and your ability to turn dollars into thousands? What about unimportant little things—your habit of reading the labels in the grocery store, your attachment to garlic, your interest in coins? What about all of these things about you? Where do inherited characteristics end?

Famous Hereditary Diseases

Huntington's disease is well-known, like its most famous sufferer. It's completely debilitating as the disease progresses, causing shaking, dementia, and early death. Woody Guthrie died at fifty-five years old.

Huntington's disease is known to be caused by a specific gene. Cystic fibrosis. Color blindness. Down Syndrome. Duchenne muscular dystrophy. Hemophilia. Sickle cell anemia. These are all famous illnesses we know to be hereditary. If we expand the search, we begin to recognize that other health conditions are hereditary, too. Heart disease tends to run in families and is related to the high blood pressure that also tends to run in families. Cancer is another. Find one member of a family who has faced it, and, sure enough, you'll find others and keep discovering more. Edward Kennedy died from brain cancer. Edward Kennedy Jr. had bone cancer at age twelve. His sister Kara had lung cancer. Cancer is so common (one man in two and one woman in three will be diagnosed with it) that it's difficult to find a family untouched by the disease. Nevertheless, it does tend to run in families.

And what about heart disease? We think of former Vice President Dick Cheney, talk show host Larry King and Bill Clinton, who underwent quadruple bypass surgery. David Letterman is the son of a man who had a heart attack at an early age. And Elizabeth Taylor and Barbara Walters, who had surgery to replace her aortic valve. More often than not, these famous sufferers had heart disease in their families.

Emotional and Psychological Diseases

What about emotional conditions like panic attacks or more run-of-the-mill anxiety? It's the same. Practitioners routinely list "family history" as one of the risk factors for anxiety disorders. With 19th-century author Henry David Thoreau proclaiming that "the mass of men lead lives of quiet desperation," we probably don't have to look far to find families that have recurrences of the disorder. Sometimes it seems practically everybody has it. Abraham Lincoln. Emily Dickinson. Of course, Van Gogh. Barbra Streisand, who forgot the lyrics to a song she was singing in a Central Park concert and reportedly suffered anxiety that the same thing would happen again. New York Yankees' second baseman Chuck Knoblauch, who got the yips and couldn't trust his throwing to first base any more (a really easy throw for a star player).

All Diseases

Let's stretch the discussion to the limit and simply say this: All disease probably relates to heredity. Why can we make such an extreme statement? Because of what we know about DNA, the substance that transmits information from one generation to another. DNA records everything. It's not just the famous instances of family tragedy like Agamemnon and other Greek myths from ancient times or the Kennedys from modern times. It's everybody, everywhere, all the time. DNA records everything and transmits everything. What if we could perfect it? What would that mean for health? For happiness? For life?

And It's Not Just Diseases, It's Everything.

DNA, this unchanging chemical link to the universe, is completely sensitive. Its influence goes not just to diseases but to things not normally classified as disease at all—your facial features, your energy level, your percolating personality, your shyness, your dislike for rutabaga. DNA is a storehouse of impressions, and not just from this life.

The problem is, we can't do much about these diseases and the DNA that controls them. That is about to change, as we get to know DNA better and find out how to manage this most delicate, most powerful blueprint at the basis of our lives. It's amazing just how powerful a recorder the DNA is. After all, it is unchanging and doesn't seem to do much of anything either. It's unnerving once you know it, or comforting if you don't mind being watched all the time.

There's the genotype and the phenotype and the epigenetics feedback loop, and the transfer RNA and messenger RNA, all described in the fanciest, most advanced scientific understanding of this chemical that you and I have running our lives. We will come to those technical terms in due time. But DNA and this knowledge of it is what makes it all physical now. We're playing the game in our own backyard, not off in some ethereal place using ideas that just don't have the clout of tangible scientific concepts no matter how much we might insist on denying this.

2

The Game of Life Is Physical

How can one substance be so important, practically God in the body? DNA is no slouch. There's no limit to what your DNA can do. Seriously. No limit. This shouldn't be that surprising. Somehow we emerge from the void to become whoever and whatever we are—Steph Curry or Katy Perry or Lady Gaga, or the guy pumping gas at the Pit Stop. We become this intricate person with bones and cells and, yup, at the heart of it all . . . DNA. It sits right at the junction point of us and the infinite pure consciousness that is the universe. That's its job. And DNA is that universe exactly. Whatever state the DNA is in, there it is transforming emptiness into fullness.

Similarly outrageous things happen in the universe, where one instance seems to have total power. Think, for instance, of a black hole, which of course amounts to thinking about a powerful inversion of absolutely nothing. A black hole cannot see itself, just as you cannot see your own face. Still, your face is there. The unbounded field at the basis of life, called the unified field in physics, also cannot see itself. But all of life comes out from there.

Consider your face again. You can see your face only as a reflection. A black hole, according to recent theory, reflects anything that comes into contact with it as a hologram.[1] When you see your face in a mirror, you see it with your mind and your eyes. When the black hole sees itself, it sees all of creation.

When someone has a hereditary disease, then, which means practically any disease at all, some part of the DNA is not being reflected fully. In Huntington's disease, one gene that is suspected to be expanded and unstable is at the root of all the shaking and dementia and decline and early death. One tiny gene!

Never Missing a Trick

As it sits there, mirror-like, the DNA is catching everything. If it could have an alternate career, it would make a great court stenographer. Smile, and it knows it. Lose your keys. The DNA jots it down. If someone does something to you, the DNA knows. Does it even record thoughts? Yes, it does. Does it put the same amount of weight on a thought as on an action? This depends on the thought, and it depends on the action. But, in its all-knowingness, it knows how to set the priorities.

Is DNA a spy, then? Of course it is, but it isn't working for a foreign power. It doesn't tell anyone else. It simply registers the behavior, and the effect of the behavior is to turn on or off genes. That is the real point. Positive influences on the genetic code move us up. Negative influences take us down. Of course, the whole set of requirements and behaviors is so complicated that you have to be one of the immortals to win at this. But the recording is relentless. Drip. Drip. Drip. Everything goes into the shimmering, fine web of your DNA.

What is this DNA that does nothing and everything at the same time?

DNA Is No Mystery—It's Chemistry

DNA has quite a job to accomplish—building muscles, bones, cells, organs, and our intricate brains. There it is, the pulsating gatekeeper between consciousness and the body, doing a job that no mere substance should be asked to do.

We know the chemistry of what happens. The structure of DNA includes combinations of four specialized molecules called "bases." Each base joins with a phosphate and sugar molecule to form a "nucleotide." If you find living tissue in anything, plant or animal, you'll probably come across these four nucleotides.

What does a cell have to do to grow from this collection of four eager wannabes into, say, you or me? This happens by the mechanism of gene expression, which occurs mainly through two processes called methylation and histone modification. Methylation is a chemical process in which a methyl group tags onto the DNA. With methylation, a single cell can grow into what we've been talking about—an eye cell or nose cell or liver cell or medulla oblongata cell, a player in a complicated organism like you or me or a tree or a wild boar or an African elephant. Methylation, as it happens, had better not mess up, or it can inappropriately silence a gene that should be operating (such as a gene that suppresses tumors).

The other player is histones. Histones are organizers. They compact the DNA into what we call a large nucleoprotein (which hearkens back to our four nucleotides, but these are now larger groups to work with). That large nucleoprotein is named "chromatin," which in turn forms the "chromosomes."

For DNA to get at its constituents and do things like replicate, transcribe, repair, and recombine, histones and DNA have to interact. Histones are regulators for processes that need to have direct access to DNA. Entrusted with so much power and influence, they actually regulate how DNA expresses itself. That's a big deal, considering the complexity of what comes out of DNA. Histones have to know what they're doing and not mess up, all of which culminates in what we call epigenetics, or the newly understood ability of DNA to express itself to our advantage (happiness and health) or disadvantage (sickness and suffering). Ah, the amazing power that resides in humble-seeming things like a little chemical called a histone.

So, what do you know now that's useful for your life? There's your chemistry. DNA consists of four nucleotides, and methyl can cap the DNA and influence its behavior. Histones glob portions of DNA together so that DNA can act on them and create things. How much does that really tell you about not getting sick? What can you do to change those things even if you want to? A lot, as it turns out, though we have to work up to all that.

DNA Actually Becomes *You*— A So-Called "Phenotype"

We now know the process where DNA becomes the ultimate product— you—or as the technical people would have it, the "phenotype." Phenotype means the observable characteristics of an organism, an intricate way to say "your body." "Pheno" comes from a Greek word that means "appearing" or "showing." So, your phenotype is the expression of your DNA that the whole world can see.

How does the DNA with its four eager nucleotides, assisted in the process by methyl and histones (a glomming together mechanism), fall into place to be you? The cycle is shown in figure 2.1.

DNA, to begin with, has all the knowledge of everything you are to become, absolutely all of it. That's a key piece that we'll come back to in our concluding thoughts at the end of the book, if not before. "All of the capability in the universe." Really? In your DNA?

GENOTYPE, PHENOTYPE, AND EPIGENETICS

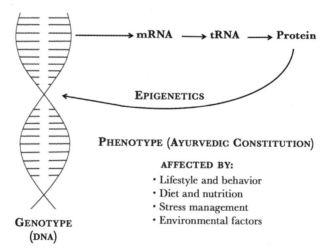

FIGURE 2.1   Epigenetics Feedback Loop

When DNA expresses that knowledge, it expresses only part of it. (Yikes. Wait a minute. What if we want it all? What would we be if we had it all?) Initially, DNA is in two strands, one from the mother and one from the father. As DNA expresses itself, the two strands separate. In the diagram, the two strands are open at the top, showing that they have separated. From the separated part of DNA a copy is formed by the process called transcription. This copy is called "messenger RNA" or just mRNA. The DNA then closes up and goes back to doing absolutely nothing. Quite the job. Minimum effort and maximum results.

The information from messenger RNA is translated by transfer RNA (tRNA), which lines up amino acids to form the protein. This is going on all the time. It's how the body works, and this process creates all the different cells in the body from those initial cells that are all the same. The resulting constitution of your body, what is known in medicine as your phenotype, emerges from your genotype, your collection of genes in a sequence that does not change. But the phenotype keeps evolving and changing and growing. If there is a problem with the phenotype, we can change it. We can fix it by acting on the phenotype to change the expression of the genotype. This is referred to as "epigenetics."

That is the portal to progress that epigenetics opens for us. That is how we can rise, and rise, and rise, and reach perfection. But I'm getting ahead of myself. For now, let's just say that biological mechanisms can turn genes on or off.

What the DNA Does Next

Meanwhile the DNA just sits there, doing almost nothing. Having stimulated a dazzling and baffling series of changes that results in the body and all our organs and our personality, the DNA rests.

As a comparison, in physics there is an unmanifest field of life called the unified field. Everything comes out of it, but it remains silent, like the black hole that reflects the whole universe as a hologram. The DNA is in charge of everything while doing nothing.

There is an Absolute level which, as we just mentioned, is called the unified field in physics. DNA represents that level, without quite being it, obviously, because it does have material form. The Absolute is pure existence, pure consciousness, and (of major import when we begin to discuss the purpose of life) pure bliss. Because it represents that unbounded eternal field that is the source of all creation, DNA is in effect a miniature universe. That's a lot of responsibility to put on a few unsuspecting chemicals.

Fortunately, the DNA is open to suggestion. As a matter of fact, it is completely, disarmingly—even alarmingly—open to suggestion. The suggestions are in that feedback loop of epigenetics. Such discussion does get us operating at deep levels of the universe. We need to understand the feedback loop to appreciate a central truth about life: DNA, once thought static, is dynamic, and even more important, we can influence what direction it goes. We can take one of the old bones of contention from ancient philosophers, whether we have free will, and drop the debate. On the physical level, we know we can change. We have free will.

3

The DNA Feedback Loop

Think of the power of this substance, the DNA. Somebody should bottle it, but it's too complicated. Complex as it is, it's individualized. My DNA isn't your DNA, isn't Katy Perry's DNA, isn't Robert De Niro's DNA. It's the blueprint at the basis of our life, barely manifest and, as much as possible, doing absolutely nothing.

Yet, in the rigmarole of life, we're doing everything to improve ourselves. We go to school. We become skilled at reading or become skilled at developing architectural blueprints for skyscrapers. Surely the DNA must change as we do all these things. We engage in self-improvement, the most popular segment of the trade book market. If we change our thinking so that we perform in new ways, there is DNA at the basis of it all.

We marry. We have children. We eat healthy, organic foods, stuff ourselves with nachos at the football game, tell the truth, tell lies, stay up too late, get up early. We live a fast-paced life and wonder why we get tired.

And there, all the time, is the DNA. What happens to it with all that we're doing? It doesn't change. Or so we thought.

"DNA Doesn't Change"—the Mistaken Old View

Your high school biology teacher, unless you happen to be a very recent high school student, told you that DNA doesn't change. Don't be too hard on him or her. DNA, in fact, does not change as far as the sequence of genes is concerned. But thanks to what we have discovered through our study of epigenetics, we have learned that the expression of DNA can be altered. The earlier concept of unchanging DNA creates a gloomy outlook on human life. It meant that if we have a gene that causes us to create a lot of fat cells without even eating much food, we have that gene, and this is all there is to it. It's not fair, but according to this view, it is what it is. Or maybe we're a bit lethargic. We'd rather watch TV or take a nap instead of finishing our projects, fixing a leaky faucet or cleaning house. Nothing is going to change that, according to this now outdated view. We're just lazy, that's all.

Enter "the DNA feedback loop" and the game changes completely.

DNA Changes Continually—The New View

To reiterate what we said earlier, DNA opens to facilitate the creation of mRNA, then closes. The mRNA is translated by tRNA. The tRNA builds the protein. Your high school biology teacher was on top of all that. *There is something else that happens* that opens the door to all kinds of wild change and progress and improvements and happiness. It's huge. It's powerful. It's life-changing. We've mentioned it before: Epigenetics. The name begins with "epi" (meaning "on top of" or "over," or "in addition to") genetics, the original makeup and phenomena of an organism.

The phenotype (the body, made up of all that protein that has come out of the DNA process) sends messages back to the DNA—called a feedback loop—which actually has incredible influence. While the sequence of genes cannot change, the genes can be turned on or off, and this amounts to the same thing as changing the DNA. Hold everything. How does it work if the DNA does change, and what gets changed is not actually the DNA itself, but the expression of the genes?

According to recent estimates, you have about 20,000 genes. They have various assigned responsibilities. Perhaps a gene is supposed to reduce inflammation in certain circumstances. Usually it's good to reduce inflammation. Turn that gene on, and the inflammation is reduced. Turn it off, and the protection isn't there. The inflammation can go on as it pleases. Even though the gene is still there and in its proper sequence, the effect is a world of difference if it is turned off instead of on. Think of a symphony of changes like that throughout the DNA. All of a sudden, the DNA itself is a secondary player. What matters is its expression.

Suppose a troupe of actors comes into the theater in street clothes—jeans, shirts, and hats, all in various colors. They go into the dressing room. Then out of the dressing room come clowns and princesses and monkeys and elephants and a ring master. They're the same people. What has changed is their *expression.*

Your body sends messages back to the DNA to turn genes on and off. This is the world of epigenetics. Not to be depressing for long, but we want to mention that you can change DNA by toxic or radiation injury, which results in mutation. Cancer comes to mind and other unfortunate possibilities if you damage the DNA. We mention these things for contrast. Changes through mutation take a long, long time. Change through epigenetics, though, comes much sooner. We can choose to change ourselves for the better.

There is hope for our situation. We're not just fatalistically locked into a life determined by DNA that does not change, because epigenetic mechanisms (with that precious feedback loop) tell us that we can change it after all. In fact, certain reliable sources estimate that epigenetic considerations determine 90 percent of life.

Does It Take a Lot to Change DNA?

The answer is no. Everything that happens to the phenotype during its lifespan changes it. You're in the womb. Your mom gets stressed out, has a fight with your dad, stays up too late, and binges on ice cream. Nestled in the womb, you feel it. Some genes may get turned on or off. If in childhood you're very happy, your mom reads you books every night, and you fall asleep to pleasant dreams, certain genes get turned on or off. The adolescence hits with a vengeance; your parents split, and you don't make the cheerleading squad. Like some kind of foreign spy system, your DNA is there recording everything because experiences turn genes on and off.

We thought we were alone. We thought we were safe. At least our lives were our own. Not quite. Thanks to epigenetics, our super sensitive DNA is keeping track of everything. Our DNA is a witness (like it or not) of everything we do. "Wax on. Wax off." Changes, changes, changes.

Epigenetics takes on a gargantuan task. All the information of what happens to the phenotype is taken to the genotype, which changes its expression. This is the process known as epigenetics. The phenotype is affected by everything that goes on in all the periods of your lifetime—prenatal, postnatal, childhood, adulthood, and a lifetime of social experiences. The phenotype is also affected by diet, nutrition, exposure to toxins, lifestyle, behavior, stress, and environment.[2-11] We would love to figure out just how all these disparate influences (too much to record in a diary or even with a film crew following us day and night) affect the expression of genes. How can we control that? Is there even hope? We might as well just eat breakfast, climb onto the A train, go to work, try to enjoy ourselves, and forget about trying to direct everything else.

A Confusing, Overwhelming Maelstrom

Genes, at least, were manageable, if you call 3.2 billion nucleotide pairs manageable. Now, with epigenetics, we are looking at constant changes in the world of those 3.2 billion nucleotide pairs. Not all of them change, if that's any consolation, during the epigenetic interplay between genes and phenotype. But your body is dynamic and ever-changing. The genes are always there as a stable base, responding to what's going on in the body.

Can we at least get a little sense of order here?

Although each aspect of living is actually complex to an unlimited degree, we can say that the following influences are the main ones that affect the body:

- Lifestyle and Behavior

- Diet and Nutrition

- Stress

- Environment

"Behavior?" That is everything you do. This is pretty complicated. "Diet and Nutrition?" This changes so much depending on where you are in the world, whether you cook at home or eat in restaurants, and so on. Still, there is some comfort in knowing that we can keep the phenotype in good health with proper principles of life and living. On the depressing side, if we don't flip on and off the right genes with these four influences, the phenotype runs into trouble and falls sick.

Even the Weather Changes You

The research is in. But think about it. Some things are probably going to affect you, maybe even deep enough to change your DNA expression, especially your diet or a condition like obesity. So will your choices about physical activity, tobacco smoking, alcohol consumption, as well as your exposure to environmental pollutants, your level of psychological stress, and working the night shift. Research has shown these things might modify epigenetic patterns.[8]

Researchers have also reported epigenetic malfunctions, by various mechanisms, in cancer as well as neurodegenerative, autoimmune, cardiovascular, and other diseases, as a result of epigenetic influences.[9]

The seasons change gene expression as well. Scientists are starting to track those influences.[10] And, no surprise, really, studies have shown that environmental stress can cause changes in your epigenetics. How about this? They're finding that we can then pass on the epigenetic alterations to our kids and even their children.[11] Bad enough that we don't get to live right. Then we're hurting those innocent descendants that we so want to cherish and nurture. Life can be hard. Researchers are starting to unravel it.

"So That's How Karma Works"

"Karma" is a hip term. Nobody really understands it, so we just toss it off now and then to be funny. "Karma ran over my dogma." We never understood it because we could never see how anything could actually be tracking it. Some religions say that a supreme god is tracking it, and he will hold us accountable on judgment day. Fine, but that day is a long way off. He might forget by then. Or he might not notice this little instance of fudging some results on the tax return.

Epigenetics changes the whole game. Karma now sits in the chemical working of our own body. Cheat in the bingo game, and the body records what you did. Have that one extra donut and the DNA is there, the tireless court reporter. It registers everything perfectly, and here is the karma part. It instantly records the full effect of everything. Nothing has to wait. We can't hope that by the time judgment day comes, the body will have forgotten all this. Our DNA registers everything, and we are accountable for every one of our actions. Do something good for ourselves or others, which means in accordance with the flowing force of evolution that is always at work, and we're healthier for it. If you sneak or cheat or, with quite good intentions, do something that is against that flowing force, the histones and methylation kick in. The all-time personal record registers it. *We can't get away with anything.*

Right there, in the feedback loop of the DNA, is that field of karma that has been pretty much a head scratcher throughout history until now. Now we see it's real. It's immediate. It's physical. In fact, it's chemical. You cannot escape it. "As you sow, so shall you reap." Or, in physics, "for every action there is an equal and opposite reaction." You'd think there'd be some loophole, but there isn't, other than avoiding life-damaging behaviors and utilizing techniques that maximize life-supporting epigenetics.

Just when things seem hopelessly, mind-numbingly complicated, nature begins to provide its own organizing solutions. At first, the emergence of epigenetics seems as much a curse as a blessing when informing us that DNA, in effect, *does* change. How are we supposed to make sense of the changes brought on by our infinite possible behaviors acting upon our 20,000 genes? Western medicine is still working to understand the full scope of this science.

But help can come from unexpected places. Enter Ayurveda, and its breadth and depth of knowledge. According to Ayurveda, impressions of actions are stored as sanskar granthi which equates with DNA which affects future actions. The factors that affect the phenotype for change are known as epigenetic factors. This whole process equates with the science of Ayurveda. More on that later. First, we want to underscore a long-overlooked point. We know where karma sits in the body.

4

Karma Is the Feedback Loop

"Karma" itself is one of those terms that took a long time making its way into everyday usage, like "chakras" (still heading that way), "yoga" (a sleeper until it enjoyed a torrent of support), or even "Facetime," "trending," or "tweets" and "widgets" (now completely commonplace terms).

Few, if any, truly know what karma means. And we haven't been fully certain that karma is real. Karma means "action." The law of karma is action and reaction. "For every action there is an equal and opposite reaction." "As you sow, so shall you reap." But people just plunge ahead with actions, with no consideration of the consequences. Or they just assume that whatever they intend to do, the karma from it will be good. If the goodness of it isn't obvious on the surface, we rationalize it. "They deserve it. I'll get good karma for being an instrument of justice." That type of reasoning.

Achilles, Lady Macbeth, the Fly on Your Computer Screen

Karma is happening all the time everywhere. It's as omnipresent as air and prana (the breath of the universe, which we'll talk about at length in a bit).

Literature is nothing but the display of karma. In *The Iliad*, from ancient Greek times, the Trojan war breaks out, death and destruction rain down from all directions, and Achilles gets buffeted and beaten. What happens to him is the consequence of his actions.

Who can think of karma without thinking of Lady Macbeth and her dark secret of having killed the king? Can the drama end without her getting her comeuppance? It cannot, because it is Shakespeare, and he is too pure a reflector of the laws of nature. Legendary Captain Ahab, obsessed with a white whale. How else can his monomania conclude? He goes to the bottom of the ocean with his hard-won prize. Vary and confound and twist it how you will, in the end karma rules. It always does.

Look in the news on any given day. It is the field of karma in our lives. "Deadly attack near UK Parliament," and we are faced with the karma of a man, of his victims, of all those who hear and know about it, of all those who don't but are alive in the universe. Action and reaction. And action spreads to the end of the universe.

A Chemical in the Body—A Little Too Close to Home

Now we are saying that good-old, abstract, ignore-me-if-you-want karma is a chemical, and it's even (theoretically) measurable. What does it mean if we are to conclude that a chemical in the body is a repository of karma? A *chemical*? We know what it means when we have epinephrine in the body, the former "adrenaline." An upsurge of power and anger and focus. Testosterone? Stand back. Estrogen? Be wary, also. Dopamine? Be careful, or you'll want more and more. Sugar (or, more technically, glucose)? That feels good. Amphetamines? You may not sleep that night, but you sure can focus on your homework.

But these localized chemicals have an effect for a few hours or a few days. Often they kick in and fade out in a moment. "I may have to fight. Oh, that was silly. No, I don't." DNA is always there and, though silent itself most of the time, always (through epigenetics) recording everything, and it's relentless and thorough.

It was pretty easy to ignore karma before we knew that it was our epigenetics feedback loop. It was so big and variated and abstract and pretty much off-the-table. You could throw it around like you might toss around "eternity" or some other half metaphysical term that might or might not have much effect.

Now that karma is a chemical—a chemical feedback loop—it changes the whole discussion. You can no longer say, "If I get away with this." You will not get away with it. You may counterbalance it or get lucky and have it turn out right. But it will be recorded, and not off in the sky somewhere. It will be recorded right in your body, and we know the chemical that will do it. D N A could be "do not ask" if it is present and working, because it is. Period. It is even working before birth and after death, but that is a topic for later chapters. Expanding the discussion beyond the present life does add a new dimension to "relentless." Death itself is no escape.

Before we go any further, some clarification is needed. You may be getting the impression that karma is a bad thing. Karma means "action." It is neither good nor bad. It is the result of action that is positive or negative. Positive action, positive results. Negative action, negative results. The choice is yours. Even if you did something negative, the situation isn't hopeless. To illustrate this point, let's consider a research study that was conducted on thirty prostate cancer patients who did not get surgery, radiation, or hormone therapy. They were put on a program that included a vegetarian diet, breathing exercises, and meditation. After three months, there were changes in the expression of more than 500 genes. The results showed that 48 genes were up-regulated and 453 genes were down-regulated. The genes that were down-regulated included disease-promoting genes with critical roles in tumor formation.[12]

In another study, meditation was shown to down-regulate the expression of genes related to stress, inflammation, and cardiovascular disease. There was up-regulation of tumor suppressor genes.[13] These studies show that negative results of previous karma can be helped by positive action combined with self-effort. Also, by meditation we get freedom from the binding influence of karma. The meditation has to be a type in which one transcends to experience the totality. A large number of other meditation techniques will not have the same effect. We'll talk more about meditation later.

Another point about good karma—it's everywhere. It's in the leadership of Abraham Lincoln that led to the Emancipation Proclamation. It's in the life of Mahatma Gandhi, who achieved India's independence by a nonviolent movement, without war. It's in everyday interactions between everyday people. We see the results of good karma—good actions—in the lives of countless individuals, and the effects of these actions emanate throughout society, the nation, and the world in a positive way.

So, in case you were scanning or skipping or not paying attention, we have said that epigenetics, the DNA feedback loop, is karma, and we know it's a lot to chew on at first. I don't see how day-to-day Western medicine is going to be able to do much with it, and I'm sure many doctors would completely agree. "Karma? I don't know much about the concept. Ask your psychic about it." Or, they might even say, "Ask an Ayurvedic expert. You'll have better luck."

And now it is time to move into the influence of that very thing—the Ayurvedic expert. We are here to go deeper and deeper into the inner workings of the body and all that plays into the feedback loop and its inevitable consequences.

Part Two

Kundalini: The Life Force

5

Fixing the DNA Is Not Just Academic

Epigenetics, from the Western point of view, is an emerging science. It's powerful, but just inching its way into existence. It deals with futures. What does it matter that Ayurveda, with all its hippie-sounding terms like chakras and prana, might actually be the means to influence the genotype in the direction of health, longevity, and whatever else is good? This matters a lot. Maybe medicine does not have to be all drugs and surgery. Maybe what we want is whatever works.

People Adjust Diet, Lifestyle, and Stress If They Can

Most of us are not in the habit of thinking about food and lifestyle as medicine. Sure, there are books with titles like "Food Is Medicine," but those are books you perhaps scan on the train when somebody leaves it on the seat. We don't take them too seriously.

But when you think about it, we are often trying to make adjustments to have a better life. Ayurveda makes a complete science of it, which, of course, is all the difference. But think about what we do. We have trouble sleeping after eating pizza late at night, so we say, "I'm going to stop eating pizza late at night." We find that stressful confrontations with our boss make us unhappy, so we try to sidestep them when we can. Ice cream makes us gain weight, so we resolve to cut back. Often we cannot do much about our environment, but we move from a less desirable house to a better one when we can.

I recognize that we actually ignore such considerations of making changes most of the time, but the stakes go up when we know that we may have a predisposition for something that will be destructive. We have a friend whose dad was an alcoholic, and it caused a lot of pain and disappointment for both the dad and the family. So the son went out of his way not to be like his dad, although often feeling inside that he was just like him and couldn't get away from it. Still, he would try to avoid drinking too much alcohol. Someone has a family history of heart disease. "So I won't smoke" is a good choice, although, if you informally survey your friends, you find that often they do smoke in spite of this history in their family.

Life comes crashing in on us despite our best intentions, but, nevertheless, we do make attempts at living right and avoiding bad influences. We just aren't very good at it, and those bad influences are often so much fun. What's wrong, then, with having guidance on diet, lifestyle, and dealing with stress that is systematic, thorough, and self-reinforcing in its results? We do it informally. Given the chance, we can do it as a science—namely through Ayurveda.

Fascinatingly, ancient Ayurveda has always looked toward diet, lifestyle, environment, and stress management as the means to elevate the physiology. It has always looked toward prevention. It has always looked toward elevating the human condition to an exalted state of health and well-being. Ayurveda aims high. It has the tools to do it. And those tools aim at the deepest level, straight at the DNA. Ayurveda goes even deeper than that infinity-straddling DNA to the energies and forces that perk up the DNA and get it to reflect the universe in the ways most satisfying and uplifting for the population.

Sometimes Ayurveda Is Heroic, the Life Saver

Of course lots of times Western medicine is obviously the hero. We think of heart bypasses and successful breast cancer surgery. There are many, many other instances, although most of them are not at the level of body chemistry in the DNA. Sometimes Ayurveda, working at the level of the DNA, is the hero. One man had a family history of colon cancer. Sure enough, in his forties, he was diagnosed with it. His brother was diagnosed with it as well. Both had successful surgery.

One of them followed a thorough regimen of Ayurveda to strengthen his overall phenotype and prevent the early onset of death. His brother did not. The one who practiced Ayurvedic techniques has been healthy for twenty years after his surgery, while his brother survived barely five years after his surgery. Sure, you might say, Ayurveda is just food and daily routine and a little sitting with the eyes closed in meditation, so how powerful could it be?

This cancer survivor is one example of Ayurveda averting disaster. Ayurvedic practices in general are a cancer preventative. When the cancer is present and surgery, chemotherapy, or radiation, singly or in combination, is recommended, that is the way to go. But for smooth sailing and cancer prevention, Ayurvedic practices are significant, as explained in the book *The Answer to Cancer* by Dr. Hari Sharma, et al.[14]

Take another example, this time heart disease. In an article published in 2012, physician Dr. Robert Schneider and his colleagues followed over a five-year period the progress of about two hundred men and women who had coronary heart disease. All of them followed the regimen of Western medicine. Half of the subjects did an Ayurvedic meditation technique.

At the end of five years, the Ayurvedic group had a 48 percent reduction in their risk of heart attack, stroke, or dying.[15] Happenstance? No. Statistically significant. Seemingly trivial, everyday Ayurvedic practices, particularly when systematic and directed at the individual, are heroic. They're game changers. They affect our life and death.

Here's another instance of Ayurveda with a man we know with a family history of heart disease. His father died at age forty-two, suddenly and in perfect health, from what was called a heart attack. His grandfather had made it to fifty before likewise collapsing and dying at work from what was called a heart attack. Our friend got the requisite EKG in his early thirties and a stress test in his fifties. He was told that all was fine. Meanwhile, he practiced Ayurvedic approaches, not for heart health but for his personal growth and achievement. At age seventy-one the docs ran a couple more scans and told him, "You have a dilated aortic root," that is, a risk of an aneurysm, almost surely the cause of death of his ancestors. And he has had the condition for a long time.

The biggest risk factor with aneurysm is high blood pressure. Because of his Ayurveda, our friend had normal blood pressure and likewise unconsciously practiced diet, daily routine, and other Ayurvedic approaches that are preventative of heart disease. He is considering surgery but, as his surgeon said, he has already broken the mold. Epigenetics, Ayurvedically-inspired, has given him a longer life.

Sometimes Ayurveda Works When Western Medicine Does Not

Take a condition like anxiety, or posttraumatic stress, or depression. Often the approach in medicine is to alleviate the symptoms rather than eliminate the cause. The cause may be lying deep in the DNA, perhaps present at birth through heredity. An antianxiety treatment alleviates the symptoms but does not operate at the epigenetic level. The anxiety remains to pop up another day.

A scientifically recommended change in lifestyle to combat stress, including learning meditation, can literally change gene expression and eliminate the disease. Often people begin meditating because they want relief from anxiety. With the practice of transcending they gain deep relaxation and recondition gene expression at a deep level. Often their symptoms disappear after their first meditation or within the first few weeks of meditating. "I tried everything," said one man in his later forties, for instance. "Nothing else worked. I suffered from anxiety since middle school. Twenty minutes of meditation and the anxiety is gone."

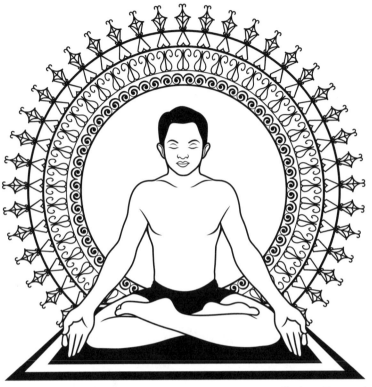

iStock.com/kumarworks

Treating the Person

We're all familiar with the medical model that diagnoses and treats disease. Ayurveda does not do that. It treats the person. It aims to make the person healthy, even if he or she has no obvious sickness. Another word for the person is the phenotype. Ayurveda balances the phenotype, sickness or no sickness.

When you consider that the phenotype reflects the DNA, and the DNA reflects the infinite, then the prospects are great for having enormous power for health and, even more important, well-being. If health is like having your car running smoothly, the real story is where you drive it. When it is running smoothly, you can focus on the trip. Likewise for the body, don't just get it running smoothly. Use it. Max it out.

Preventing and Alleviating Any Disease

Diagnosis in Ayurveda is not about discovering a disease or multiple diseases; it's about uncovering imbalances. Treatment for this, using diet, lifestyle and other modalities, is focused on restoring the body's balance. Such an approach has a number of implications:

- Rather than treating one disease (though Ayurveda can do that too), it promotes general health and well-being in a person.

- Not only do Ayurvedic practices treat known conditions, but also incipient conditions that may not yet have shown symptoms. They still show up as imbalances.

- Treatment does not need to be based on knowledge of what conditions a person is suffering from, or may suffer from in the future, from the viewpoint of Western medicine. The treatment focuses on creating good health, and conditions melt away, often before they even show symptoms.

- Ayurvedic methodologies often delay the start of conditions hidden in the DNA, such as Huntington's disease, Lou Gehrig's disease, and Alzheimer's. In fact, as we noted earlier, any disease can be delayed.

- Additionally, by improving emotional stability and happiness, Ayurveda can improve quality of life even for those who have begun to experience symptoms. For instance, a woman I know suffered from early onset Alzheimer's, and she was understandably miserable. She began Ayurvedic treatments that enabled her to experience the bliss of the Absolute at a deeper level. As a result, she became more balanced and stable inside, even though she continued to have Alzheimer's.

- Ayurveda, by restoring balance at the genetic level, also tends to lengthen life.

Operating at the Epigenetic Level Does Matter

In opening the floodgates to changing the DNA (its expression only), epigenetics is inviting medicine to discover mechanisms for working on the deep level that is the level of DNA. Western approaches, often invaluable, know only the expressed level. Ayurveda, knowing both the expressed and unexpressed levels, is even more valuable. It operates at the level of both the genotype and phenotype for a complete and holistic approach to health and well-being.

6

Ayurveda: "We've Got This."

Ayurveda has long known the unsurpassed intricacy of the human body and solved its mysteries. This science of life is comfortable not just with something as refined as DNA but with the unexpressed levels of life that direct it.

Western Medicine Trapped on the "What Is Expressed" Side of Things

What does Western medicine do in the light of the whole new ball game in which scientists who recently thought our genes were unchangeable now know from our understanding of DNA that genes can be modified in a controllable way? Some would love to leap in to perform wholesale gene replacements and save the human race. But how exactly do you replace a gene? Most discussions of gene replacement begin with a phrase "in the future" because at the moment we just can't do it. The risks of experimentation with our genes are enormous, and we basically are left contemplating our own limitations as modern scientists.

Most scientific studies of epigenetics have looked at the possibilities related to DNA methylation. It makes sense to work with something physical and palpable. Methylation, we know, changes genes. We have a good starting point then. However, once we move out of the conceptual stage, we're pretty much helpless. You don't just blow a bunch of methane onto the cell and hope it changes in a good way.

Western medicine, again quite understandably, looks at what you can see. It looks at cells, the genome (all the genes in the body form the genome) and at DNA, RNA, and nucleotide interactions . . . all pretty heady stuff. But a new player, who is actually an ancient player, has decided to join the discussion—ancient Vedic medicine, or Ayurveda, which comes in from a completely fresh direction. Instead of scrutinizing what we can see, it brings thousands of years of experience with what we can't see. Western medicine is looking ruefully at the DNA door. Ayurveda, on the other hand, holds the keys to that very door and is standing inside.

Ayurveda At Home with the Unexpressed

DNA sits comfortably on the junction point of (on the one hand) all those biochemicals and everything else that we can see and measure and (on the other hand) the infinite, unmanifest field of pure consciousness. Not in reaction to Western medicine, but from inclination and long tradition, Ayurveda intimately and thoroughly knows the other side of the game—the unmanifest. It does not have to start from scratch to figure out how to manage gene expression or discover how the DNA is influenced, but rather has a long, long history of influencing the DNA, even before anyone knew the molecular basis of heredity was going by that name.

Take the Ayurvedic tool of meditation, for instance—the process of slipping beyond the surface level to deeper and deeper levels of creation and into that unmanifest field of our transcendent selves. In the area of awareness, similar to the effect of epigenetics in the cells of the body, meditation creates a self-referral loop to the pure consciousness area of peace, bliss, energy, and power. In the process of meditation, when the mind transcends the senses, mind, intellect, and ego, and reaches the deep inner self—pure consciousness—our mind starts imbibing the properties of pure consciousness, and these are expressed in the daily activity of life.

Ayurveda, with meditation and other tools, influences and strengthens the DNA itself. At the same time, it has recommendations for operating at the holistic level to influence our lifestyle,

diet, environment, stress . . . all the known influences on the phenotype. Ayurveda can be considered the science of epigenetics cover-
ing the manifested expression of life and how to maintain our living
in proper order and how to influence the genotype for better health.
The epigenetic factors in life affect the phenotype in a positive or
negative way and indirectly affect the genetic expression in a positive
or negative way, which can be transmitted to the progeny. Ayurveda
covers both aspects of life—genetic and phenotypic—and is a comprehensive, holistic, and personalized system of health care.

To Ayurveda, Human Life Is Cosmic Life

Ayurveda means the "science of life"; "ayus" means "life" and
"veda" means "knowledge" or "science." As this science of life looks
at the process of emerging life, it begins by observing that every living creature starts life as one single cell. The fertilized embryo is
derived from the union of two germ cells—one from the male parent, which Ayurveda refers to as purusha (wholeness) and the other
from the female parent, which Ayurveda calls "prakriti" or "shakti"
(cool names, referring to power).

As long as the two cells remain separate, no reproduction
occurs, and we have no story. When they combine, the genes that
form the genetic code of an individual come with two strands, one
from each parent, representing purusha and prakriti. The strands
cannot be differentiated as to which came from the male and which
from the female. (We are stymied on this one, I guess. You'd think
you could determine this. Wouldn't a strand have the genetic code
of the one it came from?)

The DNA, as we've mentioned, represents the material equivalent of the Absolute. In Ayurveda, the qualities of the Absolute are
Sat-Chit-Anand: Pure Existence, Pure Consciousness, and Bliss.
The Absolute is the source of everything, but does not do anything
to create the universe. When the Absolute is expressed in the form
of DNA, as previously noted, we say that the human is a miniature

universe. Ayurveda operates comfortably in such an all-encompassing view of the human makeup, a view that is quite overwhelming, and rightly so, to a world attempting to know the whole thing piece by piece.

Pure Energy? Pure Being?
We've Got That in Ayurveda.

Ayurveda, not tethered to knowing only what it can measure, knows also what it can't measure directly. It sees the phenotype as physical, as energy, and as unmanifest being. These invisible possibilities raise the possibility of a sneak attack from behind the lines on everything going on in the genome. We don't have to know it from the outside. The inside will do just fine. Here is the basic Ayurvedic view of you, me, and any individual.

The human being is comprised of the following parts:

- What is Manifest

  The Objective: Our Physical body

      Physical sheath

      Energy sheath

  The Subjective: The Inner Faculty (Working Consciousness)

      Mind

      Intellect

      Chitta

      Ego

- What is Unmanifest: Our Inner Being—the Self

The Physical Body

This contains the physical sheath and the energy sheath:

    Physical Sheath: This is something Westerners can understand and relate to as the manifested body, familiar to our thinking. It takes birth, grows and develops, and finally dies. Ayurveda has a more elaborate description of its formation from the five mahabhutas, which correspond to the five spin types of quantum physics. Ayurveda also describes the primary organizing principles of the body, known as doshas, and the different human constitutional types. These topics are discussed in chapter 9.

Energy Sheath: This contains life force and energy that connects the physical body with the mind. It gives us the sensations of hunger and thirst. At the time of death, this sheath disconnects from the physical body. This energy is not visible to the average naked eye, but only to those with a special ability to see it, and is said to be visible with high-frequency photography. If Ayurveda has long known about it, we might ask, then why not help the rest of us out? Is it the person's aura? Can we manage it and work with it? For further details about the energy sheath, see chapter 7.

The three familiar elements Ayurveda includes as part of the Inner Faculty (Working Consciousness) are mind, intellect, and ego—terms you know well enough. The fourth element, unfamiliar to many Westerners, named "Chitta" is a very cool thing from the Vedic tradition. This is the storehouse of impressions. It's real mind stuff. For esoteric subjects like past lives, chitta raises a whole new world of possibilities. Intellect doesn't store anything. It just analyzes it. Chitta's warehouse is completely different. Welcome aboard. Who knows what wonders lie in there? There are lots of them—impressions from previous lives, those little bumps and twists that we would rather forget, deep inner knowledge that we never gained, but still can access . . . all kinds of things. The chitta. Who knew?

Our Inner Being—the Self as Witness

How do you squeeze our inner being to put it into a bottle? You can't. You don't see it. But it's in there witnessing everything, which sounds a lot like the silent DNA and, in fact, this silent inner being is contained within the DNA. And Ayurveda gives us hope of understanding it. Ayurveda is familiar with silence interacting with what we can see—meaning consciousness becoming matter. The unmanifest consciousness, with totality of knowledge, is manifesting on the material level as DNA.

Ayurveda *Is* the Science Above Genetics (Epigenetics)

Who is this player who comes onto the genetics playing field and claims it can handle everything? Ayurveda has an interesting resume. It deals with both the basic field (consciousness) and the expressed field (the phenotype, or the body). It has the techniques, we will see, for maintaining the body in proper order and also (the most difficult of challenges) to influence the ungainly and unapproachable genotype. It is hard to get that deep. The genotype is there shimmering at the gateway to consciousness. It doesn't change, but another "type" does, and it is the one we live by. Phenotype does change. Most drugs and chemicals don't touch the genotype. Yes, the genotype knows the chemicals are there. But it takes finesse to change the DNA expression. You have to go deep.

Ayurveda is a master of those known influences of lifestyle, diet, environment, and stress on the deepest level. Those influences affect the body, and they affect the DNA itself. That is, they affect DNA expression in ways that get transmitted to the progeny. Nobody may have expected epigenetics to take the form of that ancient science that talks about chakras, prana, body type, and a whole menu of topics not generally on the table for medical docs. But it is time for this. As the science of epigenetics, Ayurveda is a comprehensive,

holistic, and personalized system of health care that not only analyzes but treats patients on the level of the DNA (and beyond). It
builds life force in the body, the only real solution to disease. It
awakens the kundalini, to be discussed in the next chapter.

7

Kundalini: Star of the Game

In a conversation with Maharishi Mahesh Yogi, Dr. Sharma asked what kundalini is. Maharishi responded by saying "Look into DNA." This resulted in investigation into the entire energy system of the physiology, which we will now discuss. We'll enter the area of Ayurveda pertaining to those energy fields that lie within the DNA and even approach unmanifest pure consciousness. Finally we can get beyond "mere" DNA (that shimmering film that is the mirror of the infinite) to the energy fields. Ayurveda goes to those root energy fields. They're unseen. They're the basis even of DNA, which is pulsating at the doorway to the infinite. This is a large claim. Can Ayurveda really quantify and classify those elusive fields that are simply energy? Can Ayurveda sort this out? We'll give it a chance.

The human being has its manifest side, namely the body. That also includes the energy sheath. It's measurable. Ayurveda is also familiar with the subjective working consciousness—the inner faculty (mind, intellect, chitta, and ego). Finally, at the core, is the unmanifest inner being, also called Atma. (Atma is not the same thing as "the soul.") The subjective is a reflection of the unmanifest Absolute. The reflection then, dynamically within itself, becomes the physical body. First out of the subjective side is a powerful substance called prana, which is composed of the subatomic particles that create photons. (All this light at the finest level of creation is quite something to note. Sometimes people experience it directly. It is that field that becomes the highest possibility for a human—the light body. More on that later.)

Energy Sheath? Wait a Second.
Unfamiliar Territory.

"Physical body." Check. Okay. Got that. You're talking something real here. "Energy sheath?" Wait a second. This is unfamiliar territory. Western medicine does not go there, at least not much. Ayurveda does because it is beyond DNA and manages it.

Here are the players.

- Prana
- Nadis
- Chakras
- Kundalini
- Marma points

Which comes first? What is inside of what? Or are some of these things parallel to the others? We have to sort this out. The energy sheath includes all of them. Collectively, they are the energy sheath. Figure 7.1 shows the energy body.[16]

We Can Measure It

A researcher at UCLA named Dr. Valerie Hunt measured energy variations in skin areas that correspond to the positions of the chakras.[17] She found the frequencies in these areas were much higher than normal. In an interview in *Science of Mind* journal,[18] she notes the frequencies of electrical activity in those areas we can readily see and, more importantly for today's discussion, those areas that correspond to the chakras. Below is a summary of these frequencies in cycles per second (now known as Hertz).

Frequency Range of Electrical Activity in Cycles Per Second in an Electromyogram (Dr. Valerie Hunt, UCLA)[18]

Brain: 0–100 (mostly between 0-30)

Muscle: Goes up to 225

Heart: Goes up to 250

Energy with subtler and smaller amplitude

(stronger in Chakra areas): 100–1600

So the brain, which seems invisible enough for most of us, performs at 0–100 cycles per second. Pretty fast. But we can measure other frequencies that (unbeknownst to Western scientists, for the most part) go with the chakras and other energy distributing areas in the body. Those channels are there. They have to be there. Why? Because we can measure them.

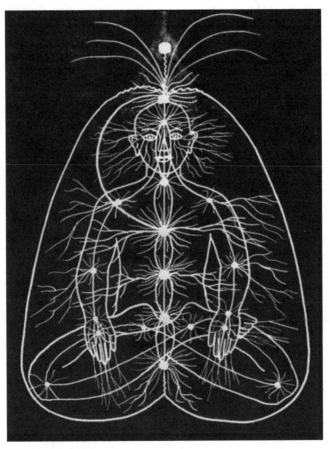

FIGURE 7.1 **Energy Body**

(Courtesy of *Ayurveda and Marma Therapy*)

And We Can Take a Picture of It.

Picture-taking has gone viral as the cell phone camera has become universal. Besides cell cameras, security cameras are everywhere. It used to be the exception to say to someone, "Smile, you're on Candid Camera." Now we can all pretty much assume that we are on camera all the time.

In the debate about human energy fields, picture taking is also sending the conversation in a new direction. "Auras are imaginary." was the old direction. Now the discussion tends more toward, "Oh, yeah. What is it we're seeing in this picture?" One source of pictures of the human energy field is the Electro Photon Imaging (EPI) camera (also known as the GDV camera), which is used in finger reading, shown in figure 7.2.[19]

Electro photon imaging, according to the website biofieldscience. org, involves stimulating and recording the electro-photonic glow around the finger. Woops, there goes the old saw that there is no aura, except in medieval paintings of the saints. Now we can take a picture of it. Figure 7.3 shows the results of finger reading.

Electro photon imaging is an advanced, digital version of Kirlian photography, which can take a picture of, well, the human aura (see figure 7.4). For years the story was, "There are no auras." Now we have pictures of them.

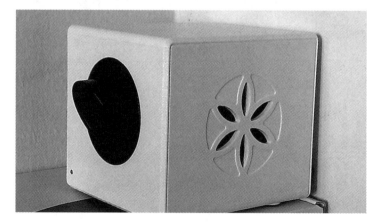

FIGURE 7.2 **EPI/GDV Camera used for Finger Reading**

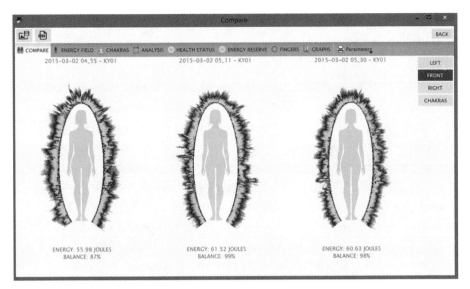

FIGURE 7.3 **Electro photon imaging of finger**

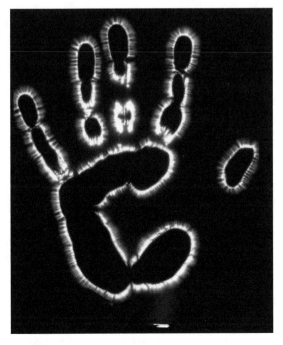

FIGURE 7.4 **Kirlian camera hand aura**

(iStock.com/Absilom)

The Primal Energy of Prana

Prana, first of all, isn't an organ in the body or anything. It is the cosmic breath. It is the life energy, the finest, finest energy in the cosmos and in us. The more of it we have working for us, the more life we have. If we're trying to figure out which comes first in these new terms, we now have a good start. Prana comes first. It's every-where—out there, and in here. When creation emerges from pure silence, the first out is prana. It creates photons, which are quanta of electromagnetic fields, and they carry energy. (Sometimes, as peo-ple experience fine levels of creation inside, they see light. That is from prana manifesting.) The finest aspect of prana is hum. After the light comes sound, which some people identify as OM, the hum of creation. Inside the body there is actually a pranic body, which is the link between the physical body and the mind. (Imagine the pos-sibilities for such a body. Is it the same as the more familiar "subtle body"? Does it live on after death?)

When creation manifests, it shows up first as prana. As shown in figure 7.5 this is the process when pure consciousness becomes matter. Vedic science knows the mechanics by which abstract pure consciousness becomes a photon or something else that you can measure. It's a huge jump that occurs. It's the mystery of the ages. Consciousness, knowing itself, becomes conscious. Pure Veda reso-nates within itself. Rik Veda represents the fundamental blueprint of the Universe, the state of pure knowledge. This is the unified value of Rishi, Devata, and Chhandas, which is also known as Sam-hita. Because it is intelligent, it knows itself (Rishi). The knowing is a process (Devata). The object of knowing is the known (Chhan-das). So, we have pure consciousness spinning within itself at high frequency and generating photons. At a later stage there is gener-ation of the five mahabhutas, corresponding to the five spin types of quantum physics, as mentioned previously. The combination of these mahabhutas generates the three doshas, vata, pitta, and kapha, which are organizing principles of nature. In the human

Consciousness and Matter

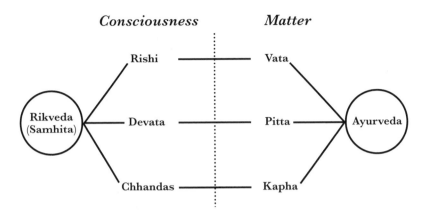

Figure 7.5 Pure Consciousness Becomes Matter

physiology, vata governs movement, transportation, and communication. Pitta governs metabolism, digestion, and transformation. Kapha governs structure and cohesion.

That's the mechanics of unmanifest consciousness becoming matter. The tendencies in the Absolute coincide with qualities in matter. They are the doshas vata, pitta, and kapha.

I realize that is a huge step with huge implications. If we can know the tendencies in nature, we can find the means to balance them. When we know how they show up in the body, we can look to reconnect ourselves with the infinite and thereby perfect the infinite in our bodies, namely, of course, DNA.

One can so easily make light of something like prana. The substance seems so small that you could just ignore it. Allow me to take a firm stand against such thinking. Prana is *almost* all powerful. Physics knows well that when the unified field begins to manifest itself, all heaven breaks loose. As pure consciousness begins vibrating within itself, it is not some sit-in-the-corner nobody. Pure consciousness vibrating within itself starts the process of the birth of the universe. Wow. So the point is, prana is a giant, the link in nature between what is manifest and unmanifest. That basic substance is very much akin to that link as we see it in the body—the DNA—except for it being even more refined and more powerful. We are standing in the presence of a giant known to Ayurveda but unknown to Western medicine.

Prana Distributors Are Nadis

Prana, as we mentioned, is energy in the body. It is the Sanskrit word for "life force" or "vital principle" of the cosmos that permeates everything in the universe. Kundalini is our individualized life force, which is not just in the spinal area but in every cell of the body. Energy resides outside the body as pure cosmic energy. When it comes into play in the body it becomes something even better. Prana is vital energy with direction. In the physiology there are five different types of prana which are distributed in different areas of the body with different functions. The kundalini is individualized life force which is not just in the spinal area but in every nucleated cell of the body. Kundalini is a force, or energy in motion. To be in motion, energy needs roads for passage. There cannot be just formless motion. We could not create human bodies, rise into the form of DNA, or do anything meaningful without channels for the force to act in. Enter the nadis.

Unlike prana, which is pure energy, and kundalini, which is the life force in the body, the nadis are actual channels in the body. Finally we have something we can almost see, or at least picture as a physical entity. Nadis are very small wire-like structures inside the body that are channels for the flow of prana and kundalini. There are 72,000 of them in the body. They distribute prana to every atom (Ah, the atom! We finally have something familiar to the West.). If some of the nadis have impurities in them, prana cannot flow there. As you can well imagine, that is not good.

You know those couch-potato days when you just can't seem to get going? It's your prana. It's not flowing through your nadis.

That's why you lack energy and feel tired. If the nadis get blocked, it's even worse. If too many of them are blocked, the prana does not reach different parts of the physiology, and we get sick.

A Few Key Nadis and What They Do

There may be 72,000 nadis (energy channels) in the body but there are three key ones: Sushumna, Ida, and Pingala. Ida and Pingala are on each side of the spine, and Sushumna is the central channel. Opening these channels is worth whatever it takes to do so. Meditation is the most proven method. Kundalini moves up the spine in every meditation and also moves within every cell. Kundalini moving up from where it rests in the lower back can open the channels like water rushing down a hill can widen a stream bed. Here are the benefits of the three key nadis:

Sushumna awakening – Sattva

The effect of awakening this nadi is positivity (sattva). We need that. Forget being down in the dumps. Fire up the sushumna nadi. It gets the breath flowing through both nostrils (for balancing your emotions and your intellect) and gets the whole brain functioning nicely. Meditation, in particular, increases the flow of prana in the sushumna nadi. I feel better just thinking about that flow.

Pingala awakening – Rajas

As this nadi opens, breath flows through your right nostril, which creates balance in the sympathetic nervous system (which controls unconscious actions and has the serious responsibility of being in charge of the fight-or-flight response). This nadi is not in charge of mental activity, but does prepare the body for physical activity, and we certainly need that. Rajas is the dynamic male principle.

Ida awakening – Tamas

With this nadi, the breath flows through the left nostril and enlivens the parasympathetic nervous system, which quiets the body and prepares it for mental work. This nervous system is in charge of rest, and we need our rest. It is the calming female principle.

PURUSHA & PRAKRITI IN CELLULAR FUNCTION

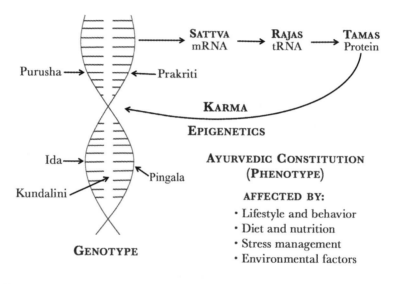

FIGURE 7.6 The Feedback Loop with Kundalini Rising

Here is where the epigenetics actually happens. As Figure 7.6 shows, when the feedback loop comes back to the cell, the DNA can open up. We want that. When the DNA opens, it can do things. Ida and pingala, shown here, are the channels through which the prana flows. Prana flowing is good. But the best thing is to get the life force of kundalini flowing. Kundalini flows up the middle of the DNA. The more cells we have with kundalini flowing, the more life force we have and the better we feel. Better yet, kundalini causes the two strands of DNA to come apart, and the expression of DNA begins.

Powerful Swirling Energy Distribution Centers Called Chakras

As for those infamous and often misunderstood chakras, they store prana (energy) in seven main centers in the area of the spinal column. Chakras are the junction point for many of those wire-like channels we just introduced, the nadis. Prana flows from the chakras to the different areas of the physiology through the nadis.

Most of the chakras are functional in the body. However, if they are not fully open and the prana does not properly flow from the lower chakras to the higher chakras, then the perception, behavior, and consciousness of the individual is not fully reflected. Blockage in a chakra will disturb its function and the function of higher chakras. This creates an imbalance in the psychophysiology of the individual and can also cause sickness and disease, since the chakras also relate to the nerve plexus, endocrine glands, and different organs and parts of the body. Disturbances in chakra functions are then manifested in corresponding areas of the body.

Since each chakra acts on a different endocrine gland, this correlation is quite wonderful because it connects the unfamiliar (these abstract, invisible chakras) with something we know and can measure. Each endocrine gland is responsible for a different function in the body. Adrenal glands, for instance, are for the fight-or-flight reaction, and the thymus gland is a key player in our precious immune system.

These chakras are whirling centers of vibrating energy, with specific frequencies associated with each of them. Lower chakras vibrate at lower frequencies (lower energy) for grosser states of consciousness. The renowned higher chakras vibrate at higher frequencies (higher energy), resulting in subtler and more refined states of consciousness.

The chakras have a color and corresponding wavelength of the visible light spectrum associated with them, from red for the lowest to violet for the highest. There is also a sound for each chakra.

These are used in sound therapies to normalize the frequency in order to improve the flow of prana. Table 7.1 shows the chakras.[20]

TABLE 7.1 **Chakras** (Adapted from: Braden G. *Awakening to Zero Point*)

Chakra	Color	Visible Light Spectrum Wavelength (Å)	Endocrine Gland	Sound
Sahasrara (Crown)	Violet	3900–4460	Pineal	Om
Ajna (Third Eye)	Indigo	4460–4640	Pituitary	Kshum
Vishuddhi (Throat)	Blue	4640–5000	Thyroid	Hum
Anahat (Heart)	Green	5000–5780	Thymus	Yum
Manipura (Navel)	Yellow	5780–5920	Pancreas	Rum
Swadhisthana (Sacral)	Orange	5920–6200	Adrenals	Vum
Mooladhara (Root)	Red	6200–7700	Gonads	Lum

The Main Purposes of Chakras

The chakras have several different purposes:

1. Primary distribution centers of energy to different parts of the physiology.

2. When associated with energy, or prana, the chakras refer to the level of magnitude of specific chakra qualities, as well as potential for diseases.

3. When associated with individualized life force—kundalini, they manifest the different outlooks.

The third purpose of manifesting our outlook, or how one perceives the world, is based on which chakra is dominant at that time.[21] Here's a brief description of the outlook for each chakra, starting with the lowest and proceeding to the higher chakras that have more refined states of consciousness:

Mooladhara chakra (Root chakra) One is aimless and does not think, is blissfully unaware of most things, wants food when hungry, and cries when there is a need.

Swadhisthana chakra (Sacral chakra) One is self-centered and tries to bring resources under their control for themselves.

Manipura chakra (Navel chakra) One is group-centered, with the group being their community, workplace, nation, etc. They have a sense of "my people" versus others.

Anahat chakra (Heart chakra) One is humanity-centered, who sees all humans as equal and seeks to approach them in the interest of all, without distinction.

Vishuddhi chakra (Throat chakra) One is a seeker and has questions in mind; for example, "What are life and death all about?" This typically happens to people later in life, when they look back on their life and ponder the ups and downs that occurred. However, it can happen early in life to those who experience traumatic events when they are young.

Ajna chakra (Third eye chakra) One is existence-centered and develops some concept in their mind about life and existence that appears to answer all their questions. If they encounter a situation that does not have an answer, they recede to the seeker level (throat chakra).

Sahasrara chakra (Crown chakra) One is fully engaged with everything in the present; there is acceptance of the past and detachment toward the future.

Each of these outlooks can be generalized in a person or can be the predominant disposition of a person. Typically, people operate at multiple chakra levels.

How to Rise Up Through the Chakras

Chakra activation occurs through the rise of the individualized life force, kundalini, which moves to higher and higher chakras until it reaches the top. The most effective and effortless process to achieve this is the self-transcending form of meditation, in which the mind reaches Pure Consciousness, creating Samadhi or Transcendental Consciousness. There are many other techniques available to activate kundalini. However in these processes the role of the teacher is more important to monitor the progress of the student.

Prana force (called Shakti) and manas Shakti (mind force) collect in the chakras. It is a good force, and we want to optimize it for health, happiness, and higher capabilities like having high-level intuition.

Distribution Centers One by One

The chakras are worth a tour. The Vedic tradition is full of information about them, including the traditional appearance of the chakras, such as four-petaled red lotus for the Mooladhara (lowest) chakra. Each one is a lotus. When the chakra is not completely open, the petals of the lotus are facing down. When kundalini rises, the petals move up and the chakra opens to allow energy, or prana, to flow freely. The appearance of the lotus becomes more refined and exalted as you move up the spine to the higher chakras.

Here is more information on the characteristics of each chakra.

Mooladhara Chakra (Root Chakra)

- Within perineal floor of men and cervix in females
- Four-petaled red lotus
- Influences excretory and reproductive organs, reproductive glands and hormonal secretion
- Associated with sacral plexus
- Directly connected to nose, sense of smell, and our animal instincts (Mahabhuta – Prithivi – Earth)
- Human evolution begins here and kundalini emerges
- Sound – Lum

Swadhisthana Chakra (Sacral Chakra)

- Two fingers above Mooladhara Chakra
- Six-petaled orange lotus
- Connected to hypogastric plexus, urinary and reproductive organs and glands
- Associated with tongue and sense of taste (Mahabhuta – Jala – Water)
- Arouses a selfish sense of ego
- Sound – Vum

Manipura Chakra (Navel Chakra)

- Associated with solar plexus – level of navel
- Ten-petaled yellow lotus
- Influences digestive process, assimilation of food and Prana

- Connected to eyes and sight (Mahabhuta – Tejas – Fire)
- Consciousness at this level still bound by grosser level of existence, sensualities, ambitions and greed
- Sound – Rum

Anahat Chakra (Heart Chakra)

- Proximity to heart; connected to cardiac plexus, heart, respiration, and thymus
- Twelve-petaled green lotus
- Responsible for emotions of love/hate, compassion/cruelty, etc.
- Connected to sense of touch and hands (Mahabhuta – Vayu – Air)
- Sound – Yum

Vishuddhi Chakra (Throat Chakra)

- Middle of throat
- Sixteen-petaled blue lotus
- Associated with cervical plexus and thyroid gland
- Maintains purity of body and mind
- Connected to ears, sense of hearing, throat and speech (Mahabhuta – Akasha – Space)
- Arouses acceptance of adversities in life, mental balance, and sensitivity to needs of others
- Sound—Hum

Ajna Chakra (Third Eye Chakra)

- Top of spinal cord at medulla oblongata

- Two-petaled indigo lotus

- Mainly concerned with higher intelligence

- Corresponds to pituitary gland

- Command center: Manas Shakti becomes more predominant; veiling power of Prana Shakti decreases

- Operates in conjunction with reticulo-activating system, medulla oblongata, and pineal gland

- It is third eye, through which whole subtle world can be perceived

- It is gateway to liberation

- When kundalini passes beyond Ajna, duality and ego cease to exist

- Sound - Kshum

Sahasrara Chakra (Crown Chakra)

- Crown of the head

- One thousand-petaled violet lotus

- When activated by kundalini, it is highest experience of human evolution

- Sound – Om

Other Distributors: The Marma Points

As if chakras and nadis are not enough, one other key way emerges for enlivening those pre-DNA, purely energy parts of our system. They are the marma points. Marma points are 108 primary points on the physical body that reflect prana or life force on the surface of the body. Marmas connect to the chakras (7) and nadis (72,000) throughout the body.[16,22] Marma points have traditionally been considered so important that there is a martial art, kalari, whose main purpose is to protect the marma points. Kalari originated in Kerala, India, and is one of the oldest existing martial arts in the world.

I know I'm bringing up marma points seemingly at the last minute, but they are no slouches. Marmas are the points, when injured, that may be life-threatening. Marmas are not superficial landmarks on the body surface, but deep-seated, vitally important physio-anatomical structures. The knowledge of marma is the oldest hidden treasure of Vedic surgical skill.

Many ancient saints got the knowledge of marma and practiced this knowledge for the betterment of suffering humanity. The marma points affect the parts of the body you can see—the tissues and organs. They can be invaluable when the need arises, because they can relieve pain.

What else can they do?

> Kindle energy
>
> Cleanse the body of toxins
>
> Calm the mind and balance the emotions
>
> Act as a curative and supportive treatment

If they do so much good, how do we get them to work for us?

Working on Marma Points: Asanas, Breathing, and Gems

Here are some therapies that work nicely on the marma points:

- Massage, pressure, herbs, color, gems, crystals, yantras, and metals (gold for vata, silver for pitta, and bronze or copper for kapha)

- Asanas (yoga positions) – Help to clear and energize marmas

- Pranayama (breathing exercises) – Increase flow of prana through chakras, nadis, and marmas

- Mantras – Facilitate flow of prana through marmas and create protective shield (kavach)

Do a few asanas for stability in those energy fields. Practice some gentle breathing to soothe the energy channels. Meditate to dive below the surface of the mind into the consciousness that flows in those energy fields. The first two are preparation for the meditation, which is the true power. In meditation, because of the presence of pure consciousness (which gives rise to the energy fields and ultimately to the body), kundalini awakens and flows in the body. Energy channels open up. The theory of flowing energy fields becomes reality.

Ojas—Getting the Message Across

We have energy in prana, the energy of the universe. We have channels for the energy in the body, the nadis. We have chakras, the distribution centers. These are all behind the scenes, deeper than the deep . . . that is, deeper than DNA. The question is, how do these abstract energy phenomena get the message across to something we all accept as real, namely the DNA.

We need a carrier, kind of a UPS of the body. Something has to get the message from that energy body we didn't even know we had to that body of flesh and blood we do know we have. It has to be a substance, not just another energy field. And we do have this. It's called "ojas." It's the master coordinator between consciousness and the physiology and mind and body.

How do we access this? By doing all the things that allow us to uplift the genome, namely by pursuing a healthy lifestyle and diet, minimizing stress, and creating a healthy environment. Diet would seem to be an especially big player here because ojas is actually the end-product of perfect digestion and metabolism. Such perfection might sound difficult to attain, but, if we do reach this goal, we receive ojas. It governs all those body doshas we've spoken of—vata, pitta, and kapha—all three, which represents the great power of ojas. Ojas can balance them, attuning us to the universe.

The following list summarizes the factors that increase ojas. Increasing ojas and avoiding reduction of ojas are central in restoring health and preventing illness.

Factors that Increase Ojas

- **Consciousness** – one's level of consciousness

- **Happiness**

- **Good digestion**

- **Food factors**
  Nourishing, easily-digested foods
  Mode of preparation
  Eating environment

- **Positivity in feelings, speech, behavior**—love and joy

- **Panchakarma** (purification therapies)

- **Rasayana** (rejuvenation therapies)

On the level of our bodies, ojas nourishes and sustains the tissue transformations, which raises us to higher and higher levels of health. We feel better, see better, taste better, just generally have a bounce in our step. To help keep us on the upside, it provides stability (blessed, anxiety-preventing stability) and enhances the immune system. What more does this actual substance do? It gives strength, contentment, and good digestion. Overall, it promotes balanced growth in the body.

All these good effects come from ojas taking our rising kundalini and transforming that abstract force into something physical that the body can recognize and appreciate.

The game is taking a new turn. What game do I mean? The life game. The game of fixing ourselves. The game of finding balance. The game of ending disease. And more. Ayurveda can wake up these long-neglected channels and points and put them into service. Can it really do that? Can it wake up channels and points that turn prana, the primal energy of the universe, into life force in our bodies—the force that the master coordinator (ojas) can take to our DNA?

And who is the king of those life forces? It's kundalini. Come out and take a bow, kundalini. You deserve our recognition. If we are going to unravel the mysteries of the light body, what it can do, and what it cannot, we are going to have to pass through kundalini.

8

Spotlight on Kundalini

Kundalini is The Show. It is what all the other invisible channels in the body are there to distribute. It has been misunderstood and misrepresented, but understand it for what it truly is, and it becomes the pinnacle.

Misunderstanding of the Life Force

Kundalini has often been misunderstood. A "coiled snake at the base of the spine" hardly denotes something positive and beneficial. Its literal meaning in Sanskrit does not convey a clear explanation of what it is. The sheer invisibility has not helped it gain recognition, either. When we cannot see or measure something, we tend either to believe it is not there or to make up myths about it. After all, there is nothing to hold us in check. "Breathe this way. It will fix your kundalini." "Avoid sex and you will store kundalini." "Sit with your back straight." "Sit in lotus." Truths and half-truths and non-truths abound.

The Grand Readjustment—It's Not Just at the Base of the Spine

One important distinction is that kundalini is not energy. It is individualized life force, and it is enormously powerful. Prana is energy—formless, primal energy, and, as mentioned, it is everywhere.

As a human body takes shape out of the interplay of tendencies in nature, the body has the ability to transform prana into something powerful in the body that is no longer energy but is a force. That force is kundalini. It is our energy in action within the body. It is awesome and exalted.

Neophytes speak of kundalini as energy at the base of the spine. We now know this force is only useful when put into motion by the wonder of a human body. A second misapprehension is that kundalini is only at the base of the spine or, when successfully expressed, rises up the spine. What is the truth of it? The reality is that kundalini is in the DNA of every nucleated cell in the body, all 3.0 trillion of them. Having the life force confined to just a small area along the spine would be very limiting. How much could it do there, especially if half the time it was blocked and barely making it up the spine at all? See it as distributed throughout the body though, and suddenly it rises to superstar status, and such is the status it deserves.

In All Its Glory, the Life Force

The force that prana becomes when it becomes kundalini is, in fact, nothing short of the life force itself. When it gives us life in the form of a life force, it is not giving us some barely useful force that just gets us through the day. It is not *just* that. When given the chance, it rises more and more in expression and gets all our senses working better and better, lends freshness and appreciation to our perspective and, as will be explained later, begins to bring the qualifier "supernormal" to otherwise ordinary senses.

We Get Sick If It Is Not There

"What do I care about kundalini? Leave that for the New Agers." I can hear it now. There's a simple answer. If the kundalini is blocked, our health is blocked. With blocked kundalini, prana does not reach our tissues, and those tissues begin to lose strength and function. We don't feel that good, and things can go from bad to worse. If you pump up the kundalini artificially when it is blocked, it goes sideways and causes problems. If you like a positive view, the more kundalini we have producing more ojas, the more bounce we have in our step and the more gleam in our eye.

If you consider our picture of the DNA (Figure 7.6—The Feedback Loop with Kundalini Rising), that special empty space in the center is where the kundalini rises up. It goes through individual cells, and also goes up the spine and through the chakras. All the energy merges with that all-powerful source of creation, pure consciousness. The rise of kundalini is the measure of enlightenment. Epigenetics brings the possibility of revolutionizing the body and individual cells with this kundalini flowing right through the silent heart of things. Consciousness expresses fully in the nervous system, and it changes the structure and function of the nervous system.

Forget all the trendy everyday uses of "kundalini." Let "kundalini" rise up to its exalted position. This precious life force is everywhere in the body in every nucleated cell. Get it fully expressed in your body and you are living the primal energy of the universe, that which creates everything, living it lively within your own skin.

When we discern the overall makeup of the body, including that unseen energy on the other side of DNA, and begin to flip all the right genes on and all the wrong ones off, we have no better instrument for doing so than that masterful kundalini.

9

Ayurveda *Is* Epigenetics

It's impressive that the genome, with its billions of nucleotide pairs, has been completely mapped. A map of the genome is a logical starting point for epigenetic treatment. Find the offending gene and change its expression. This is challenging work that is now in its infancy.

The newcomer, Ayurveda, also scopes out the physiology down to the finest level, using different tools. In its long tradition, Ayurveda knows how consciousness turns into the body and, as tendencies in nature combine, into body type. If you know the body type, you know a lot about the person. You can guess correctly his or her proclivities ("You can't resist chocolate," "You would prefer not to participate" [for just about anything], "You have hair-trigger temper," etc.) . . . often to the person's wide-eyed surprise.

Ayurveda, this ancient player new to the epigenetics stage, does not map the genome to know you intimately. But it distinguishes the body type in Ayurvedic terms. The steps for doing so are quite elaborate, quite reliable and accurate when done thoroughly, and are now beginning to be validated by Western scientific practice as well.[23-32] By the way, body type stems from deeper levels of the universe than even the DNA level. In the next chapter, we begin to scope out those intimate inner levels.

Making a Body Out of, Basically, Nothing

In keeping with its ability to know everything from the inside, Ayurveda begins with consciousness itself, and then unfolds what happens as the consciousness becomes your genome. Ayurveda's name for a fully developed map of "you" is the psychophysiological human constitution, or "prakriti." If you understand your map and any imbalances in your constitution, you can then make changes to create better health and eliminate disease. Ayurveda describes two types of prakriti: Birth prakriti (janma prakriti) and psychophysiological constitution (body prakriti or deha prakriti). Birth prakriti does not change and is the foundation of the psychophysiological constitution or body prakriti, which changes and is dynamic. If the psychophysiological constitution or body prakriti is out of balance, it is known as vikriti. Birth prakriti equates with genotype and body prakriti equates with phenotype. Ayurveda manages the body prakriti (phenotype) through recommendations for lifestyle and behavior, diet and nutrition, stress management, and environmental influences. These factors affect the birth prakriti (genotype) by changing its expression, thus Ayurveda equates with what is currently known as epigenetics.

As consciousness comes onto the material level, it takes the form of the five Mahabhutas, or the five spin types of quantum physics. This is fundamental to knowing the body. If we know the body's basic constituents from the source, then in treatment we can get those basic elements re-attuned to their source to fully reflect the infinite. This is powerful, just as the genetic structure is fundamental and powerful.

The five Mahabhutas in Ayurveda are:

- Akasha (Space)

- Vayu (Air)

- Tejas (Fire)

- Jala (Water)

- Prithivi (Earth)

Some people are spacey. Some are well grounded. Some are fiery. These five elements become human bodies. You're probably not used to thinking of the body as the expression of space, air, fire, water, and earth. You think of it as cells and blood vessels, or maybe as atoms and molecules. But it truly is made up of the five elements.

Physicist John Hagelin, PhD, has found correlations between these five elements and the five fundamental "spin types" of quantum physics, as the unified field manifests into energy and matter. See table 9.1. In quantum physics spin is an intrinsic property of the two classes of elementary particles, known as bosons and fermions. These differ in spin. Bosons have an integer spin, i.e., 0, 1, etc. Fermions have a half integer spin, i.e., $\frac{1}{2}$, $\frac{3}{2}$, etc. This difference in spin type results in fundamental differences in behavior. Bosons create coherent states, whereas fermions do not. Both are necessary in the structure of the universe, to create uniformity and differences. At an underlying level, bosons and fermions are the basic building blocks of nature. These spin types correlate with the five mahabhutas.[33-35]

TABLE 9.1 **The Five Mahabhutas or 'Great Elements' and the Five Spin Types of Modern Physics**

Five Mahabhutas	Five Spin Types
Akasha (Space)	Spin 2 = Graviton (Gravity)
Vayu (Air)	Spin $\frac{3}{2}$ = Gravitino
Tejas (Fire)	Spin 1 = Force Fields (Electromagnetism)
Jala (Water)	Spin $\frac{1}{2}$ = Matter Fields
Prithivi (Earth)	Spin 0 = Higgs Fields Invisible energy fields.

Space, air, fire, water, and earth sound like folklore. Such an analysis of the body isn't folklore once we view it in terms of quantum physics. The Spin 2 graviton, for instance, is responsible for the heady concept of space-time curvature. Hence it has a neat correlation with the Vedic Mahabhuta of Akasha (space). All five spin types are shown in table 9.2.

The Spin 1 force fields, seeming to have nothing to do with your body or anyone else's, are the champions of electromagnetism, a key player in light, heat, and chemical transformations. Now it is beginning to sound more like the body, and it is. The Mahabhuta Tejas (fire), which is related to digestion, is also essential to sight. We've previously mentioned photons, the fundamental particles of visible light. Well, they're Spin 1.

And there is the famous Higgs boson with spin 0, known for being quite mysterious. Some call it the "God particle." The Higgs boson is responsible for giving particles their mass. What are we without mass? "Nothing" is right. So the Higgs boson corresponds with the Mahabhuta Prithivi (earth). As we anticipate the rest of this discussion of the structure of the human body, we begin to get a sense of what happens from the interplay of these five fields—namely, everything we know at any observable level, including the body.

TABLE 9.2   **The Five Spin Types from Modern Physics and the Five Mahabhutas from Ayurveda**

Spin Type	Mahabhuta	Correlation
Spin 2 = Graviton (gravity)	Akasha (Space)	Space-time curvature
Spin 3/2 = Gravitino	Vayu (Air)	A candidate for dark matter
Spin 1 = Force fields (Electromagnetism)	Tejas (Fire)	Responsible for light (photons), heat, and chemical transformations
Spin 1/2 = Matter fields	Jala (Water)	Elementary Fermion particles
Spin 0 = Higgs fields	Prithivi (Earth)	Give particles their mass

Fundamental Energies Mingle

From the five Mahabhutas comes another essential intermingling, leading us ultimately toward the Ayurvedic equivalent of the genome. The doshas, as mentioned previously, are the primary organizing principles of the body, known as vata, pitta, and kapha. Know them, manage them, and the world is your oyster.

Vata is formed from the combination of the space and air Mahabhutas. Pitta is formed from the combination of fire and water. Kapha is formed from water and earth. Once again, there is a direct correlation with the field of quantum physics. Dr. Hagelin has correlated the formation of the three doshas from the five Mahabhutas with the formation of the three superfields from the five spin types. See table 9.3.

These pulsating, nearly infinite energy fields combine at a profound level of the body, in fact at the DNA level, to create three operating principles in your body and everyone else's.

TABLE 9.3 **The Three Doshas (As Combinations of the Five Mahabhutas) and the Three Superfields (As Combinations of the Five Spin Types)**

Mahabhutas combine to form *Doshas*		*Spin Types* combine to form *Superfields*	
Akasha (Space) and Vayu (Air)	→ Vata	Spin 2 and Spin $^{3}/_{2}$	→ Gravity
Tejas (Fire) and Jala (Water)	→ Pitta	Spin 1 and Spin $^{1}/_{2}$	→ Gauge
Jala (Water) and Prithivi (Earth)	→ Kapha	Spin $^{1}/_{2}$ and Spin 0	→ Matter

Ayurveda, from long experience and from the cognitions of seers throughout time, knows the qualities of each of these fundamental energies operating in the body (or should we say, in the phenotype). Table 9.4 gives a summary of these.

These doshas govern the entire body. Table 9.5 lists the functions of each dosha.

> **Vata** represents motion and flow. It controls the movement of your lungs when you breathe, the beating of your heart, and the flow of blood through your blood vessels. In Ayurveda, channels such as your blood vessels are called shrotas.
>
> **Pitta** is associated with the fire element known as Agni. Pitta regulates digestion and directs all metabolic activities and biochemical reactions in the body.
>
> **Kapha** is associated with the dhatus, which are principles that uphold the formation of bodily tissues like muscle. Kapha is responsible for proper body structure and biological strength.

TABLE 9.4 **Qualities of Vata, Pitta, and Kapha**

Qualities of Vata	Qualities of Pitta	Qualities of Kapha
Cold	Warm	Cold
Light	Light	Heavy
Quick	Sharp	Oily
Dry	Slightly oily	Sweet
Moving	Fluid	Steady
Minute	Hot taste	Slow
Rough		Soft
Leads the other doshas		Sticky

TABLE 9.5 **Doshas at Work in the Body**

Dosha	Associated with	Functions
Vata	Shrotas	Transportation
		Movement
		Communication
Pitta	Agni	Metabolism
		Digestion
		Transformation
Kapha	Dhatus	Structure
		Cohesion

Being Becoming Matter

Try to do it yourself. Take your own consciousness, be silent, and have matter emerge. Good luck with that. Nature does it, and there is a logical sequence to it. Consciousness is three-tendencies-in-one even as it sits silent within itself. Consciousness, first of all, knows itself. It is intelligence, so it knows things. When it is pure consciousness, though, what is there for it to know? Just itself. (Matter isn't emerging yet. But just wait.) See figure 9.1 for a visual show of what we're saying here. The knower (consciousness) looks at itself (the known) and this is a process – the process of knowing. After a number of intermediate steps, there is formation of the Mahabhutas: space, air, fire, water, and earth.

When consciousness is pure intelligence (the knower), it correlates with space and air. This is still pretty abstract. There is the teeniest bit of matter there, but let's move on. The process of knowing correlates with the elements of fire and water. When it is the known object of its own perception, it correlates with water and earth.

Voila. Mystery of the ages exposed. Consciousness becomes matter—the five Mahabhutas, or, more acceptable in our scientific era, the five spin types. The next step is that the five elements correspond with the three physiological principles in the body—vata, pitta, and kapha, as shown in the figure.

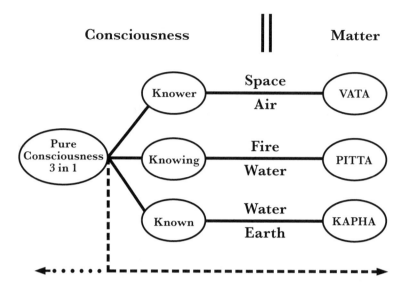

FIGURE 9.1 Consciousness Becomes Matter

Once we have the three doshas and see them as pure consciousness expressed in the body, we're ready for everything. If the objective for health is to get our body reflecting the universe, and if we know vata, pitta, and kapha in the body, we can then balance them to get them reflecting their source, which is pure consciousness.

We have the setup for analyzing the body down to its deepest levels.

Know Thyself, Know Thy Body Type

Western medicine is beginning to identify neurotransmitters (brain chemicals that transmit information throughout the brain and body) that coincide with each of the doshas:[23]

> **Kapha** – High histamine, which is associated with the allergic response. You are probably familiar with antihistamines, which you take when you want to tamp down the allergic response and open your sinuses. It fits with this body type made from water and earth, as shown for example by "runny nose."

Vata – High acetylcholine, a chemical that stimulates muscle movement. This fits with a body type that tends toward high activity. Acetylcholine is also involved with attention and memory.

Pitta – High catecholamines, which includes powerhouses like epinephrine (the former adrenaline; Pittas are fighters) and dopamine (the addiction chemical).

There is no parallel in Western medicine for the Ayurvedic concept of human constitutional types. However, a Western medicine analysis in terms of biochemistry is helpful in delineating the differences in Ayurvedic constitutions.

Table 9.6 shows how body frame, hair, memory, aging, and all kinds of other things vary with the different body types. The more detailed information we have, the more we can look at features of someone's body (like being thin or heat-intolerant) and relate these to a body type. And if we know a body type, we can help to keep the body in balance (meaning avoiding imbalances that are the cause of disease), using tools that can change epigenetic expression by adjusting lifestyle, diet, environment, plus using some special tools like meditation.

TABLE 9.6 **Distinguishing Features of the Three Body Types**

Features	Vata	Pitta	Kapha
Body frame	Thin	Medium	Broad
Body build and musculature	Weakly developed	Moderate	Well developed
Skin	Dry and rough	Soft, thin, with tendency for moles, acne and freckles	Smooth and firm, clear complexion
Hair	Dry, thin, coarse and prone to breaks	Thin, soft, oily, early graying	Thick, smooth and firm

(continued)

TABLE 9.6 Distinguishing Features of the Three Body Types *(con't)*

Weight gain	Recalcitrant	Fluctuating	Tendency to obesity
Food and bowel habits	Frequent, variable and irregular	Higher capacity for food and water consumption	Low digestive capacity and stable food habits
Movements and physical activities	Excessive and quick	Moderate and precise	Less mobile
Tolerance for weather	Cold intolerant	Heat intolerant	Endurance for both
Disease resistance and healing capacity	Poor	Good	Excellent
Metabolism of toxic substances	Moderate	Quick	Poor
Communication	Talkative	Sharp, incisive communication with analytical abilities	Less vocal with good communication skills
Initiation capabilities	Quick, responsive and enthusiastic	Moderate, upon conviction and understanding	Slow to initiate new things
Memory	Quick at grasping and poor retention	Moderate grasping and retention	Slow grasping and good retention
Aging	Fast	Moderate	Slow
Disease predisposition/ poor prognosis	Developmental, neurological, dementia, movement and speech disorders, arrhythmias	Ulcer, bleeding disorders, skin diseases	Obesity, diabetes, atherosclerotic conditions

(Content of table is from "Whole genome expression and biochemical correlates of extreme constitutional types defined in Ayurveda" by Prasher B, Negi S, Aggarwal S, et al. *J Transl Med* 2008;6:48. doi:10.1186/1479-5876-6-48)

When Ayurvedic experts know an individual's body type, they can have an inkling of diseases people are likely to get. For example, kapha people, who tend to carry a bit more weight than others, are at risk for heart disease. There is strong relation of risk factors (diabetes, hypertension, dyslipidemia), insulin resistance, and inflammatory markers with vata-kapha prakriti and kapha prakriti.[27]

Analysis of body type according to Ayurvedic medicine is a reliable indicator of the risks people face in their health. In a clinical study, maximum platelet aggregation, which is indicative of susceptibility for blood clotting, was highest among individuals with vata-pitta prakriti, and they responded better to lower doses of aspirin which helps prevent clotting. Another clinical study showed that the incidence of Parkinson's disease is highest in those individuals with vata prakriti. This study may be helpful in identifying those who are susceptible to Parkinson's and delaying the onset of symptoms or slowing the disease progression. In another clinical study, biochemical parameters were studied and the results showed that kapha individuals have high risk factors for heart disease, whereas pitta individuals have high values of hemoglobin and red blood cells and vata individuals have high serum prolactin levels and high prothrombin time. Prolactin is important for both male and female reproductive health, and high prothrombin time means the blood takes too long to form a clot. This can be seen in liver disease, vitamin K deficiency, or clotting factor deficiency. The science of epigenetics, still feeling its way, can also identify risks in a few instances. Looking at the two perspectives together, we see the reliable conclusions from Ayurveda beginning to be borne out by analysis at the genetic level.[23-32] Prakriti (body type) analysis is epigenetic analysis.

Ayurveda, having identified the risk by knowing the prakriti, is expert in working at those finest levels of the body to make the body work better, even at its best. It all starts with prana, the finest breath of creation and also of your body. Ayurveda, coming from a basis in the infinite that underlies even that pulsating DNA at the basis of life, identifies the fundamental energy principles in the body. Vata. Pitta. Kapha. It then identifies, in exhaustive detail, the qualities and behaviors of each, and the diseases that arise when one or more is out of balance. The following tables give details on the doshas.

TABLE 9.7 **Seven Types of Individual Physiological Constitutions (Prakriti)**

Vata
Pitta
Kapha
Vata—Pitta
Vata—Kapha
Pitta—Kapha
Vata—Pitta—Kapha

TABLE 9.8 **The Three Doshas—Functions**

VATA	**PITTA**	**KAPHA**
• Respiration	• Appetite	• Strength
• Elimination	• Digestion	• Stability
• Touch	• Heat	• Weight
• Hearing	• Sight	• Generosity
• Thought	• Contentment	• Healing
• Speech	• Endocrine functions	• Growth
• Biological rhythms		• Taste
		• Smell

TABLE 9.9 **Signs of Balanced Doshas**

BALANCED VATA	BALANCED PITTA	BALANCED KAPHA
• Exhilaration	• Contentment	• Affection
• Alertness	• Courage, dignity	• Generosity
• Normal formation of tissues	• Sharp intellect	• Stable mind
• Normal elimination	• Normal heat and thirst	• Normal joints
• Sound sleep	• Good digestion	• Muscle strength
	• Lustrous complexion	• Vitality

TABLE 9.10 **Symptoms of Imbalanced Doshas**

IMBALANCED VATA	IMBALANCED PITTA	IMBALANCED KAPHA
• Dry or rough skin	• Rashes	• Oily skin
• Insomnia	• Inflammatory skin diseases	• Excessive sleep
• Constipation	• Ulcerative colitis	• Lethargy
• Common fatigue (non-specific cause)	• Visual problems	• Mental dullness
• Tension headache	• Peptic ulcer	• Slow digestion
• Intolerant to cold	• Heartburn	• Sinus congestion
• Degenerative arthritis	• Excess body heat	• Nasal allergies
• Underweight	• Premature graying or baldness	• Asthma
• Anxiety, worry	• Hostility	• Cysts and other growths
• Irritable bowel syndrome	• Irritability	• Obesity

TABLE 9.11 **Characteristics of Ayurvedic Constitutional Types**

	Ayurvedic Constitution		
	Vata	**Pitta**	**Kapha**
Mental activity	quick mind, restless	sharp intellect	calm, steady, stable
Memory	short-term is best	good general memory	long-term is best
Become afraid	very easily	easily	slowly
Learn new things	very quickly	quickly	slowly
React to stress/ problems	excite very quickly, worry a lot	anger easily, quick temper	slow to get irritated
Amount of hair	average	thinning	thick
Type of hair	dry	medium	oily
Skin	dry, rough	soft, medium oily	oily, moist
Weather	aversion to cold	aversion to hot	aversion to damp, cool
Sleep	light, interrupted (4-6 hours)	sound, medium length (6-8 hours)	sound, heavy, long (> 8 hours)
Dreams	fearful, flying, running, jumping	anger, fiery, violent	water, clouds, relationships, romance
Weight	thin, hard to gain	medium weight	heavy, easy to gain
Walk	fast, quickly	slowly, changing	steady, non-changing
Exercise tolerance	low	medium	high
Endurance	poor	good	excellent
Strength	poor	good	excellent
Hunger	irregular	sharp, needs food	can easily miss meals

(continued)

TABLE 9.11 **Characteristics of Ayurvedic Constitutional Types** *(Con't)*

Food and drink	prefer warm	prefer cold	prefer warm and dry
Eat	quickly	medium speed	slowly
Elimination	dry, hard, constipation	many, soft to normal	heavy, slow, thick, regular
Financial	doesn't save, spends quickly	saves, but big spender	saves regularly, accumulates wealth

Here is a sophisticated way to know, not the DNA in this case, but the finest physiological makeup of the body, nevertheless. With our knowledge of body types, we can use it to fix people's health problems—to relieve pain, break up blockages in the body, and clear up our thinking. Not only does prakriti help in treating disease; it often helps where Western medicine is handcuffed because, as we've said of Ayurveda, it goes to those root energy fields that are the basis even of that subtlest expressed substance, DNA. So it helps in prevention of illness. More than that, it helps in enriching the life of a perfectly healthy person. It can perk up the fine energy fields of the body. It is a gateway to those fine energy fields, the shapers of the DNA.

There are factors that interfere with all that potential for progress. We need to identify the enemy in this fight for health and beyond to have a clear-cut opponent so we know where we are waging the fight. We could say the enemy is disease or imbalance of our body, and surely it is. But the best name for the enemy in the time we live is probably "stress." Let's have at it. If we're going to rearrange ourselves back into the fundamental patterns of the universe and turn our kundalini loose to our infinite delight and ecstasy, we're going to do it by overcoming nothing less than the enemy—stress itself.

Part Three

Diet, Lifestyle, and Meditation

10

Stress: The Enemy

Diet, lifestyle, environment . . . they all help to liberate us from our limitations as mere humans, and we see their power in the ensuing chapters. But we need to know the enemy. What they are liberating us from is stress. Once an unknown player in the whole game of evolution, progress, and the search for liberation, stress has now become a major player. Conquer stress and you have conquered most health problems. However, that conquest seems all but impossible.

What Is Stress?

Stress clogs the nadis. Free the system of stress and the nadis open up and kundalini flows. Of course, we do not generally define stress. Everybody knows what this condition is, right? You don't have to *define* it. Feelings of stress occur when someone honks at you when you are letting a pedestrian cross in front of you. It's a result of the experience of waiting all morning to go to your favorite Thai restaurant for curried noodles, only to get there and find out it's closed for some reason. It's what you feel when you go out of your way to pick up the kids from school just to please your wife, and had informed her that you would do this, only to have her berate you for not telling her you were picking them up.

It's the big things that happen to us that create stress in our lives—for instance when we are having problems with our kids, even when our kids have grown up. It happens when we are sick or when we are told things like:

- "You're fired."

- "We need to talk."

- "You've been hacked."

- "Usually that recovery procedure works. Sorry."

- "This is the IRS."

- "Are you sitting down? I need to tell you something."

- "Don't worry yet. It doesn't look too serious."

In addition to the major stressful events in life, the small conflicts, disputes, and inconveniences that occur in day-to-day living can drag life down, and hinder progress and growth.

- Your bicycle chain snaps.

- You can't find your briefcase.

- Someone pays you a compliment like, "You look better today," which makes you wonder how you looked yesterday.

- You notice a big stain on your favorite blouse.

- You hit every red light on the way to work.

Big things. Little things. Earth-shaking things. Everyday things. Sometimes things that are upsetting for no obvious reason. Stress comes relentlessly seeking us out, and finding us.

Everyone thinks they know what stress is. Obviously. Of course. "Don't ask me to explain the obvious." If someone does take the time to look it up, he or she might find something like this from the website helpguide.org, "Stress is your body's way of responding to any kind of demand or threat. When you sense danger—whether it's real or imagined—the body's defenses kick into high gear in a rapid, automatic process known as the "fight-or-flight" reaction, or the *stress response*."

Twists in the Nervous System

How does the fight-or-flight response clog the nadis? Stress is a reaction to what happens when something is an overload. In popular parlance, we say we're "fried" or we're "toast." The fight-or-flight response does not usually itself cause an overload, but an excessive fight-or-flight response can do this.

Some overload causes twists in the nervous system. Nerve impulses cannot flow smoothly through that area. Nadis get blocked. Kundalini cannot get through. Such a definition is helpful, and hopeful, from a medical point of view. While, yes, we can manage the environment to attempt to lower stress, we have an easier job if we just work close to home—on the body.

How Do You Manage It?

To manage stress, Ayurveda recommends proper living and proper knowledge of life, as well as yoga, pranayama (breathing exercises), meditation, whole-body massage, Ayurvedic psychotherapy, and herbs. Here again is a potpourri of approaches, and each contributes something. If stress is actual kinks in the system, then whole-body massage sounds like a reasonable approach, but it may not go deep enough. The sequence we often recommend can be a relief:

1. Yoga asanas

2. Pranayama

3. Meditation

Then engage in as many of the other approaches as you can—a proper diet, a comfortable environment, a good and healthy lifestyle. Mix in some good influences from Ashwagandha, precious gems, and anything else on the list.

An encouraging sign comes from the perspective that sees stress as physical. You can dissolve it. The more you dissolve it, the more flexible you become inside, and the less you accumulate it from the next challenging event. In fact, any of the aforementioned instances causing stress, from small things like lost keys to larger things like being ill or losing your job, need not be a stressor in themselves. They are a stressful situation only if they cause an overload. The more powerful you become inside the more kundalini is flowing—the less the episodes cause stress.

Can We Rid Ourselves of Stress Altogether?

Certainly that seems impossible. Stress is as commonplace as Kleenex. If you want to find some common ground with a stranger, just begin talking about health problems or the economy or the way the government always seems to end up shooting itself in the foot. You know you're going to find something in common—problems, complaints, misery, stress.

Realistically, when you think about it, no, you cannot escape stress any more than you can escape life itself. Plunge into life and you meet unexpected reversals and, hence, overloads. Don't plunge into it and it's even worse. The inertia weighs on you. Life is dynamic and insists that you be progressive. You accumulate stress.

However, as we think about the body arising from pure consciousness (which is perfect), we begin to have a glimmer of hope. If it is possible to become more and more flexible, and thereby less responsive to stress, couldn't you become totally flexible and thence completely free from stress? Well, yes, that is the ultimate goal.

Stress, Epigenetics, and DNA

In our modern understanding, where we cannot change genes but can change gene expression, removing stress means changing gene expression in the positive direction. You do not even have to know what that positive direction is. The body figures it out as the kundalini flows through the nadis and into the manifest level, the DNA. The beneficial genes turn on; the not-so-beneficial ones turn off.

We understand what the enemy stress does to us. It blocks us. It makes us sick. When we do something wrong, we block some nadis too. If we do this over and over, we sink more and more into the baser levels of life. This is a physical and automatic response and not pleasant at all.

What can we do about behavior to keep our nadis open?

11

Is It Worth Being Good?

Someone can tell us, "Here are the rules for correct behavior," but we might prefer not to follow them. You might respond, by saying, "This doesn't work for me or my lifestyle." Yet on the other hand, we cannot escape the fact that the tireless recorder, DNA, is recording our every thought, word, and deed. It's enough to make us throw up our hands in despair, or simply ignore this situation altogether.

As we have seen earlier, our lifestyle, diet, stress levels, and environment are not merely innocent happenstance, but in fact influence us at our deepest level—in our gene expression. Are you out of work and out of sorts and watching a lot of TV and drinking too much beer? This can suppress kundalini flow. Do you find that your desires are heading in a negative direction instead of toward progress, peace, and happiness for your family? Your pranic flow will then take a hit. Remember, the DNA does not miss anything. It's an in-house spy, and a relentless one at that.

It is better for the deep levels of the body for us to have uplifting thoughts. But uplifting thoughts alone are not transforming. Don't put too much responsibility on them. Rules of behavior alone are not going to establish flowing, rambunctious, deeply energizing kundalini. They need help.

Guidelines for Lining Up with the Five Spin Types

If we think of rules of behavior as guidelines for lining up with the spin types of nature for better health and well-being, and not as rigid moral precepts, the behavioral guidelines then become more palatable. The Vedic tradition has laid aside all pretense that behavioral guidelines are strictly ethical do's and don'ts. They have practical value in life and are seen as recommendations to achieve good health and emotional balance. Here are the guidelines for behavior from the book *Ayurvedic Healing* by Sharma and Clark.[36]

Behavioral Rasayanas

Behaviors and attitudes to be maximized are:

> Love
>
> Compassion
>
> Speech that uplifts people
>
> Cleanliness
>
> Charity and regular donation
>
> Religious observance
>
> Respect towards teachers and elders
>
> Being positive
>
> Moderation and self-control, especially with regard to alcohol and sex
>
> Simplicity

Behaviors and attitudes to be avoided are:

> Anger
>
> Violence
>
> Harsh or hurtful speech
>
> Conceit
>
> Speaking ill of others behind their backs
>
> Egotism

Dishonesty

Coveting another's spouse or wealth

The list is just a general invitation to knowledge for enhancing health and well-being. These are not severe, heavily enforced, Puritanical morals. They're guidelines to help you feel better . . . deep down, way deep down, where the epigenetics feedback loop is flipping genes on and off all day long.

Social Behavior Is Not the Primary Means to Good Health

First of all, be advised that considerations about our behavior toward others are not the primary technique for opening the nadis and becoming a pure reflector of the infinite unboundedness. Recommendations for having positive feelings toward others and having the goal of being a good person are supplemental. If you don't have something more powerful for opening your nadis, such as meditation, pranayama, and yoga asanas and some truly elevating diet, you're just frustrating yourself if you go around trying to be virtuous all the time. The behavioral recommendations are just good advice to keep good relationships and self-respect. Telling yourself, "Don't get angry" is good if you have enough distance in a difficult situation to remind yourself of that. More powerful than telling yourself, though, is having inner stability in your physiology. Having good health is primary.

But remember, it's not the end of the world if you show a little wrath. You don't have to go around constantly reminding yourself to stifle any flare-ups. All that concentrating on self-control and suppressing yourself causes that one thing we most hate—feelings of extreme stress. These recommended behavioral rasayanas are part of a team of DNA enhancement techniques, but they don't work well in isolation. They're in a support role.

How Do We Know We're Helping Our DNA?

You can sort of tell when you are improving yourself, depending on how many nadis you have open already. If you're addictive, eating the wrong foods, or skipping meals altogether, your system probably isn't tuned in to the effect of one more event of acting well. It's an entropy thing. If the amount of disorder is high, one more stir of the pot doesn't make much difference. If it's low, then each stroke shows up. So, if you've been virtuous and respectful to your mom and dad and eating at the right times, you may notice a wave of good feeling when you say something nice to someone.

Measuring the effect of the right behavior is not so much a strict science as a feeling and an art. How good does it feel to help an old lady with her groceries or be polite to a counter clerk? It feels good, but we don't have to take our blood pressure before and after to demonstrate that the behavior has helped us. Be easy about it. Behavior is just one more way to open our shrotas (channels like the veins and arteries in the body) so that the kundalini can flow through the nadis, those channels for flow of energy.

If we get our DNA working pretty nicely, the good behavior in your lifestyle should be a simple thing to help keep things going well. That's all. It's certainly better not to do some outrageously nasty thing. On the other hand, don't be so scrupulous about your habits that you won't even watch a movie that contains some negativity. Be easy about these kinds of choices. Trying to always do the right thing is good for your DNA but not altogether a game changer.

On the other hand, doing things you know to be wrong registers on the DNA, becomes stressful, and wreaks havoc. You don't get away with it. That notion is a concept from the twentieth century and before. Now, in the epigenetics era, we realize you don't get away with anything. The approach to your diet is about the same. Eat right, but you don't have to be a food faddist, especially the self-righteous, hypercritical kind.

12

Diet: Can It Flip the Genes?

If we want to attune ourselves to the mahabhutas (the five elements), diet is a great candidate. Some foods, obviously, are hot. We're talking spicy-hot. Had any Mexican chilis lately? They increase pitta in the body, and that is not good if you have enough pitta already. On the other hand, some foods are cooling. Cucumbers are famous for their cooling effect. But if you're a slowed-down kapha type, cold cucumbers may not be your best choice.

Certain Ayurvedic advisors will tell you in great detail how to manage your diet to suit your body type. Often the recommendations can have radically beneficial effects. For instance, we knew a fellow who loved spicy food and could not give it up. He was a pitta body type, and the spicy food was causing health issues for him. When he finally dropped the spicy food altogether and began eating cooling foods, his health and happiness sprang back.

Food can be extremely attractive to faddists, who often become so sold on them because of their own benefits from eating certain things that they become proselytizers (and sometimes unpopular in the process). You will hear: "Eat raw." "Don't eat dairy." "Eat vegetarian." "Eat only fruit." "Don't eat at night." "Eat only at night." "Eat this kind of garlic because it's more healthy." "Drink wine. It gets rid of free radicals." "Don't eat nightshades." "Eat raw fish." "Only eat vegan." It's interesting and helpful to learn about the latest medical research about what's good or bad for us. But try to use good judgment about food choices and don't rely on advice from people who seem to have little common sense about nutrition.

Diet can definitely be a powerful means to attune oneself to the universe. If the name of the game is to get the body to be a pure reflector of the energy of the universe, diet has to be a player. But managing diet can become so cumbersome as to be a source of stress in itself.

Recommendations for Food by Body Type

Once you know your body type, eating according to recommendations based on your body type will help to keep you in balance with the universe. For example, *Ayurvedic Healing* by Sharma and Clark[36] recommends for a vata-pacifying diet to eat naturally sweet foods like fruits; grains such as rice and wheat; cooked vegetables such as beets, carrots, asparagus, and sweet potatoes; boiled milk, ghee, fresh yogurt, nuts, most oils; and meats such as chicken, turkey, and seafood. The sweet taste is the foundation of a vata-pacifying diet, and provides an opening you can drive a truck through. But I don't think it means binging on Snickers bars all day.

For a pitta-pacifying diet, eat foods that are cooling, foods that are sweet, foods that are bitter, and foods that are astringent. Both cooked and raw foods can be eaten. Eat sweet cherries, pomegranates, mangos, and plums. Avoid sour ones. Eat lots of coconut. That's just the recommendations for fruits. There are other recommendations, of course, for nuts, proteins, starches, and other categories.

To complete the picture, there are specifications for a kapha-pacifying diet, too. It is recommended that people with this body type eat foods that are light, dry, spicy, and easy to digest. The food should be eaten warm or hot. Here are some examples of advice for this diet:

- reduce use of milk

- eat lighter fruits, such as apples and pears

- for a sweetener, honey is considered excellent for pacifying kapha

- eating all types of beans is fine

- reduce all nuts

- eating most grains is fine, especially barley and millet

- eating spices like ginger, black pepper, and turmeric, etc. is good

- eating vegetables is fine, except for tomatoes, cucumbers, okra, and sweet potatoes

We definitely can move our feedback loop in the right direction by eating the foods that are right for our body type.

Location, Time of Day, Season of the Year

Coordinating diet by body type can seem rather confusing, and sometimes it is. We are told to eat honey for a kapha diet. For vata, eat sweet things, but don't eat honey (which is sweet, isn't it?). For pitta, oh, go look it up.

Diet changes with the seasons, too, and the part of the world where you're living. And the time of day. You might ask, "Is it okay to eat a banana at 4:00 in the afternoon in Hong Kong if you're a vata body type?" Sometimes it's hard to figure it all out. However, as with following any map, you can map out your food preferences, and your body can begin to resonate with the whole thing. By the way, it varies with your age, too.

Maybe Just Keep Your Diet Simple

Many people may begin with an aggressive approach to following a complicated Ayurvedic diet, but end up over time choosing a more simplified version. A pitta body type may just habitually avoid the chilis and not eat much yogurt either. A vata may find that it is quite delightful to eat soothing, creamy foods and will migrate in that direction.

What if you're a mixed dosha? You can evolve an appropriate diet for that, too. If you're a pitta-kapha, for instance, avoid too much chili, but eat some because it's good for your kapha side.

Often the test is just how you feel. If you overdo things, before long your body rebels, and eventually you learn. Maybe you're pitta but you love chilis. Before you knew about your body type, you ate plenty of chilis and blamed your headaches on overwork or staying up too late. When you become familiar with your body type, though, you can begin to make the small adjustments. Over time they'll add up to big adjustments.

As complex and confusing as food choices are, your diet is a primary influence on your physiology. A healthy diet based on body type can be a technique for evolution in itself. Some people plan their day around a healthy lunch supported on both sides by an appropriate breakfast and a light supper, all cooked at home and served in a soothing environment. Some even see such a routine as essential and perfectly normal. On the other hand, in the modern world, some people cannot cook at home and have to take meals when they can. Even then, it's important to make some accommodations for your body type.

Diet, by itself, will not transform an individual's human body into a pure reflector of the consciousness inside. Diet alone can't do this. If you live a stressful life, don't get enough sleep, and violate behavioral recommendations, your good diet will just be a bit of salve to your many wounds. Still, it's a big player, and it's good to have diet in play. It helps open the nadis, for sure. So does where you live.

13

You Are Where You Live

Your house. Your city. Your country. How much choice do we have in these things? Can your house block your nadis? Can the country you live in set up your feedback loop so that you feel oppressed and aggressive? Can your father's country where he lived do this as well? What about your great-grandmother's country, even though you never lived there? How sensitive a recorder is the DNA? How good is its memory? What can you do about such outside influences now?

Environment Is a Big Influence

Vastu shastra, meaning "science of architecture," is a system of principles that is part of the ancient Vedic sciences. Vastu deals with architecture and interior design for optimal health. It has rules that follow the five elements (the five mahabhutas: space, air, fire, water, and earth) and the four cardinal directions (north, south, east, and west). Vastu construction gives knowledge regarding the axis, shape, and topography of the land. For the house, it discusses the optimal direction for the entrance and the best interior design. According to Vastu recommendations, a front door facing east is considered auspicious and most beneficial. In the bedroom, suggestions are provided for the location of the bed, electrical items, heavy furniture, and so forth. Recommendations are also given for the direction of the head while sleeping. Adherence to vastu principles will enable:

1. A harmonious and relaxing atmosphere

2. Promotion of well-being, happiness, and peace

3. Maintenance of balance and orderliness in life

4. Improvement of concentration and proper decision-making for family work and business

5. Putting people in harmony with the home and the home in harmony with the universe

Research studies show the effect of direction. Animal studies found that the neurons in the thalamus and hippocampus change with direction and place.[37] With a north orientation, animals were restless and aggressive. They had elevated noradrenaline (a hormone reflecting an aggressive state), so nobody was just imagining their aggressiveness. It was seen in their hormones, which means it was affecting the DNA. Animals with an east orientation looked calm and quiet. Animals with a south or west orientation had minimal changes. How could environment have so much effect? It is nature at a deep level, and we cannot escape being in nature.

But what about humans? It shows up in sleeping. Vastu recommends sleeping with your head in an east orientation for good health. A north orientation is considered to have destructive influences. A study found that humans lying down with a north orientation had irritation and confusion of thinking, and their hormones bore that out. They had elevated plasma cortisol and serum cholinesterase (these chemicals become elevated with stress). Not convinced? Their brain waves in the alpha and beta rhythms damped down. Alpha brain waves are associated with relaxation, and beta brain waves are seen with the waking state of consciousness. In an east orientation humans felt peaceful and relaxed. South and west orientation had minimal effect on humans.[38]

Sound and Music

Vibrations affect us. Sound and music are vibrational energy. Cells vibrate dynamically. They transmit information via harmonic wave motion. The list below summarizes some striking studies about plants.[39–41] If things don't interest or alarm you until they're about humans, these studies are nevertheless striking.

Effect of Sound and Music on Plants

- Nadeshwaram music

  Vigorous plant growth

  Early flowering

  More yield of grain

- Low-note broadcast

  17.3 percent increased yield of corn

- Plant growth

  Positive reaction to Ravi Shankar and Bach

  Negative reaction to acid rock

Sound and music affect us as humans also, and not just our moods as you might expect.[42] They affect blood pressure and more, as shown below:

Effect of Sound and Music on Humans

- Physiological effects

  Decreases blood pressure, heart rate, respiratory rate

  Decreases myocardial oxygen demand

  Lowers cortisol levels and interleukin-6 levels

- Premature infants

  Increases weight gain

  Increases oxygen saturation

- Hospitalized patients

  Reduces amount of sedatives/analgesics

  Reduces anxiety

- Benefits lessening of acute and chronic pain

- Improves sleep

- Improves quality and length of life in dying patients

How does music have these measured physiological effects? Here are three proposed mechanisms of action for the effects of music:

- Affects brain directly: acts on limbic system → opiates – regulates emotional responses

- Mediated by nitric oxide and opiate processes in the central nervous system and peripheral nervous system

- Cellular level—intracellular structures vibrate dynamically

Environment. We cannot escape it, and we cannot escape its influence (its very real influence, which happens, yes, at the epigenetic level and hence, on the DNA).

Tables 13.1 and 13.2 show a comparison in support of our case that environment influences us at the deepest level. Table 13.1 shows that Vedic sounds of Sama Veda decreased cancer cell growth. No such luck when the cells were in the presence of hard rock music (much as I hate to think that everybody's mother was right when she said, "Can you please turn that music down? It's giving me a headache.")

As with everything else, we're free to speculate and stick to our own preconceptions in the absence of scientific evidence. Even with such evidence we are free to think as we want, but the case becomes ever more compelling that, yes, the environment influences us at the deepest level. We cannot just "tough it out" and breeze through our environment unfazed. The DNA is too good at what it does. It picks up on everything, and our DNA expression changes accordingly.

TABLE 13.1 **Sound of Sama Veda and Decreased Cancer Cell Growth**[42]

Sound-Induced Changes in Cell Growth: No Sound vs. Sound of Sama Veda			
Tissue/Organ	**Classification**	**Cell Line**	**% Change**
Brain	Malignant glioma	U251-MG	−25.3
Breast	Adenocarcinoma	MCF7	−16.9
Colon	Adenocarcinoma	HT29	−19.9
Lung	Carcinoma	A549	−22.4
Skin	Malignant melanoma	RPMI 7951	−12.4
Skin	Normal	NHDF	−13.9

Sound of Sama Veda decreased growth in all cell lines ($p < 0.005$, ANOVA) as compared to no music.

TABLE 13.2 **Hard Rock Music and Increased Cancer Cell Growth**[42]

Sound-Induced Changes in Cell Growth: No Sound vs. Hard Rock Music			
Tissue/Organ	**Classification**	**Cell Line**	**% Change**
Brain	Malignant glioma	U251-MG	22.1
Breast	Adenocarcinoma	MCF7	26.9
Colon	Adenocarcinoma	HT29	14.1
Lung	Carcinoma	A549	6.1
Skin	Malignant melanoma	RPMI 7951	Only 1 experiment
Skin	Normal	NHDF	10.2

In presence of hard rock music (AC/DC, "Back in Black") growth of cells was increased ($p < 0.03$, ANOVA) compared to no music.

Even Your Grandfather's Environment Affects You

The sun, the moon, and the stars are huge celestial bodies that are putting out vibrations. Those vibrations reach our planet. Of course they affect us. For example, as the full moon affects the ocean tides, it similarly affects our human emotions. What can we do to maximize these distant influences or dodge the bad influences? Even our ancestors' environments affect us, and we know they lived in some rough places. Look deep into a family's history and ask why they moved to a new environment. Sometimes the answer is, "If we had stayed where we were, we might have been killed." This is stress, and welcome to the clogged nadis you still have because of it.

Suppose your great grandfather lived on the Ohio frontier, with the constant threat of being killed by either the native inhabitants or wild animals. He stored all that in his DNA. Some of that you now have. Or your grandfather worked in an asbestos plant. You were never exposed to it. Your DNA still has some of the effects.

It's always nice to provide scientific verification. Studies have found that environmental toxins such as fungicides and pesticides promoted epigenetic transgenerational inheritance of reproductive disease. Other studies have found that a large number of different types of toxicants (plastics, hydrocarbons, DDT) promoted transgenerational inheritance of disease from obesity to cancer. In animal studies environmental stress has shown epigenetic transgenerational inheritance. Indeed stress gets passed from generation to generation.[11]

Turn It Around

On the one hand, it's discouraging how much the environment can damage your DNA. On the other hand, you can get an advantage by living in a supportive and healthy environment. You don't have to do anything. You don't have to create some positive mood. Just be there. Live in an east-facing house, preferably built according to the ancient principles of Vedic architecture. When you work face the east. Don't have large bodies of water to your south. Sleep with your head to the east. Play harmonious music when you choose to listen, or have it playing quietly in the house when you're away. Environment is working all the time on that recorder at the basis of your life, your DNA.

The biggest epigenetic tools are stress management and careful management of your individual lifestyle, diet, and environment. You can't just ignore them by putting mind over matter and expect to be happy, successful, and healthy. You might be able to ignore them in your thinking mind, but your ultra-sensitive DNA ignores nothing. You will get the effects. You may not acknowledge them intellectually until, say, you get cancer or age a little faster.

We've said, quite emphatically, that the effects of lifestyle, diet, and environment on the DNA are not sufficient in themselves to turn everything around for us. They have a big influence, make no mistake about this. But transformational? That's a tall order. They're a good start, and they're pleasant to do, too. Eat right. Live in the right place. Talk nicely to people. And what more can you do? There are additional Ayurvedic tools you can apply directly to yourself to get the feedback loop working advantageously.

14

Basic Ayurveda

It is of no use knowing that the energy fields are there unless we can actually turn them to advantage. Otherwise, it's just frustrating. What does knowing about prana, kundalini, and chakras bring in itself? Instant ecstasy, insight, and enlightenment? Just knowing intellectually that they are there does not change anything. We need to affect them on a physical level. To get the energies flowing, we need meditation, asanas, pranayama, vibrational therapies, and a virtual symphony of uplifting practices that can refresh our DNA and transform our lives.

You can get bewildered at all the approaches, and you can't trust the recommendations of your friends, either. Someone will say, "I've got this great yoga position for headaches." "Hot yoga. It's the best." But someone else responds with, "I do cold yoga." "No other massage loosens you up like this massage." Yes, there are many approaches that affect the gene level. Everything affects it. You can affect it in a positive way.

The more we hear about the *possibilities* for working with deeper levels of the body, the more we want to know how to do it. Often not scientifically tested until recently, alternative approaches sometimes have a credibility problem with the public. But they have proven results, too, and potent techniques for getting beneath the surface of the body.

Alternative Approaches—Lining Up with Fundamental Energies

Ayurveda, as we stated earlier, dares to venture into that ethereal space where the unmanifest becomes manifest. First you were nothing, then a sperm and an egg, and now you're you. Ayurveda suggests that one of the first steps is the emergence of the five elements, the mahabhutas: space, air, fire, water, and earth. Then those elements combine in a few known and manageable ways to become the three doshas—vata, pitta, and kapha—which form the individual's constitution.

Notice how the body is now connected with something more fundamental (primary tendencies in the universe), which then connect with the Absolute. In managing the flow of fundamental tendencies in the body, we can restore our harmony with the universe. It's not like that just happens, but when we get it right about body type, we're getting it right about the genome. We hook up with the universal level of life, more than we did before, and we feel better than we did before we had this knowledge.

Credibility: Scientific Studies of Ayurveda

Ayurveda has thousands of years of clinical experience to back it up. Now there are a rapidly increasing number of scientific studies in the field of Ayurveda using modern scientific methodologies. The results support what the ancient Vedic texts have been saying for thousands of years. Research has shown that genes involved in the stress response, inflammation, and cardiovascular disease were generally found to be reduced in expression in subjects who practice Transcendental Meditation. In contrast, the levels of expression of two tumor suppressor genes were found to be increased.[13] In a randomized controlled trial including 201 black men and women with coronary heart disease, the Transcendental Meditation program significantly reduced risk for mortality, myocardial infarction, and stroke. These changes were associated with lower blood pressure and psychosocial stress factors.[15] A study of individuals with different Ayurvedic constitutions showed different levels of neurohormones specific to each constitutional type.[23] Other studies have found differences in genome expression and biochemical parameters in different Ayurvedic constitutional types.[24]

More studies can be found in the following books: *Scientific Basis of Ayurvedic Therapies* by Dr. L. C. Mishra (New York: CRC Press, 2004),[43] *Rasayana: Ayurvedic Herbs for Longevity and Rejuvenation* by Dr. H. S. Puri (London: Taylor & Francis, 2003),[44] and *Ayurvedic Healing* by Dr. Hari Sharma and Dr. Christopher Clark (London: Singing Dragon, 2012).[36]

No mere patsy, alternative medicine is establishing a foothold by providing research studies of its own. Meditation, in particular, has been leading the way. And now there is research on the genetic effects of alternative approaches.

Gene Expression and Prostate Cancer

A study was conducted on thirty men with low-risk prostate cancer who declined surgery, radiation, and hormone therapy. They routinely engaged in the following practices:

> Breathing exercises
>
> Meditation
>
> Low-fat, whole-food, plant-based diet
>
> Moderate exercise

The results were good, and included:

> Lower blood pressure
>
> Lower LDL cholesterol (the bad cholesterol)
>
> Lower prostate-specific antigen (this is increased in prostate cancer)
>
> Improvement in psychological functioning
>
> Lower weight

Best of all, the study found a change in activity of 500 genes, with 48 genes turned on (up-regulated), and 453 genes turned off (down-regulated). These down-regulated genes included disease-promoting genes with a critical role in tumor formation.[12]

Chromosomes and Aging: Telomeres

A telomere is the segment at the end of a chromosome. Shortened telomeres are correlated with a shorter lifespan. The telomerase enzyme stabilizes telomere length. Researchers have now confirmed what has been suspected. Stress shortens telomeres, and hence, life. The good news is that intensive changes in lifestyle and nutrition were found to increase the length of telomeres. Also, research showed telomerase activity and telomere length improve with mind-body skills training (such as yoga and meditation). Yes. That is what is needed more and more in Ayurveda—scientific validation. Even better, validation is coming at the level of the gene and the genome.[45-49]

Track Record Helping with Cancer

Alternative approaches have proven helpful with cancer. We're not saying they replace surgery or radiation or chemotherapy; nor are we saying one should forgo them in favor of a vegetarian diet and regular yoga asanas. We're saying they help, and that much seems obvious. Likewise, if people are happier, they generate fewer negative neuropeptides, and negative neuropeptides weaken the immune system. There are reliable research studies on ways Ayurveda can help with cancer.

Meditation helps with stress reduction, enhances energy, and positively affects overall health, including decrease in anxiety, depression, and pain.[50,51] Ayurveda has preparations known as rasayanas that promote longevity, stamina, immunity, and overall well-being. One of these rasayanas is an herbal mixture known as Maharishi Amrit Kalash (MAK), which has been researched extensively in laboratory, animal, and clinical settings, and has been found to have a wide range of significant beneficial properties. MAK prevented and treated breast cancer, prevented metastasis of lung cancer, and caused nervous system tumor cells (neuroblastoma) to regain normal cell functioning. It also enhanced the effect of a nerve growth factor in causing morphological differentiation of nervous system tumor cells (pheochromocytoma), inhibited the growth of skin cancer cells (melanoma), and inhibited liver cancer. In clinical studies, MAK has been shown to reduce the side effects of chemotherapy, without reducing the efficacy of the cancer treatment. For details of these studies, consult Dr. Sharma's chapter on "Contemporary Ayurveda."[52]

There are other herbs and spices that have shown beneficial properties. For example, ashwagandha has been heavily researched and found to have a wide range of beneficial effects. It is antioxidant, anti-inflammatory, anti-stress, and anti-cancer. Its anti-cancer properties include enhancing immunity, inducing apoptosis (cell death), and inhibiting the growth of new blood vessels and the spread of cancer. Ashwagandha also sensitizes tumors to radiation and anti-cancer drugs while protecting normal cells.[53]

Turmeric is a spice that has been extensively researched and shown to have a broad range of beneficial properties. It is more DNA-protective than powerful antioxidants such as vitamin E and beta-carotene. It stimulates glutathione-S-transferase, a detoxifying enzyme that protects against cancer. Turmeric protects against inflammation, inhibits precancerous colon lesions, suppresses colon cancer, and inhibits the growth of breast cancer cell lines.[14,54] In brief, Ayurveda is helpful for cancer patients in the following ways:[36, 42-44, 55-59]

Improves quality of life

Acts as an adjuvant or co-therapy with chemotherapy, radiation, post-surgical care

Minimizes side effects of conventional cancer therapies

Slows growth of cancer when chemotherapy and
radiation are contraindicated

Involves rasayana therapy, which is rejuvenation
therapy that improves comfort and quality of life

In dealing with cancer, Ayurveda does find itself in a support
role, though it is more than equipped to take the lead when the
topic is prevention. Nevertheless, even after the onset of cancer,
Ayurveda has proven its mettle.

Ayurveda Can Be a Powerful Ally in Combatting Cancer

What happens when we focus the expertise of Ayurveda on the
management of one of the most troubling diseases of our time, the
one resistant to almost everything—namely, of course, cancer?
Cancer is an important example because it is a disease of the cell.
It is DNA gone haywire. Through epigenetics the expression of
DNA can be changed. This is what Ayurveda does. Ayurveda has
been epigenetics in action for thousands of years. The discoveries
of modern epigenetics are the science behind the theories and practices of Ayurvedic medicine. Here, in compressed form, are a series
of powerful techniques for helping in the management of cancer.
Some you may do as recommended by your physician. Some, if not
all, are at least harmless, if not downright beneficial, and therefore
can be practiced along with conventional cancer treatments.

- Meditation, pranayama (breathing exercises), and yoga

- Working with the energy system—chakras, nadis, marma

- Sound therapy—a therapy based on vibration. As shown
  in chapter 13, a study found that the sound of Sama Veda
  decreased growth in cancer cell lines as compared to no
  music. In contrast, hard rock music (AC/DC, "Back in

Black") increased growth of cancer cells as compared to no music.[42]

- Ojas enhancement and removal of ama. Good digestion and other Ayurvedic practices naturally enhance ojas, the oily substance your doctor has never heard of. It's the communicator between the energy levels of the body and the manifest levels, as discussed in an earlier chapter. Ama is sludge in the system. Sludge blocks the flow of kundalini. More about Ama in the next section.

- Suitable nutrition, and proper digestion and elimination

   This includes dietary advice according to the constitution of the individual and taking into consideration the disturbances in the physiology. Ayurvedic diet and digestion is a comprehensive and elaborate system which is personalized according to the patient's condition.

   Diet should be anti-inflammatory; immune-enhancing; nonacidic; aim for proper ratio of omega-3 and omega-6 fatty acids; contain no refined sugar.

- Proper sleep

- Use of natural products that improve immunity and have anti-inflammatory, anti-angiogenesis, pro-apoptotic, and anti-tumor properties. Some of these are ashwagandha, amla, guduchi, shatavari, triphala, turmeric, grapeseed extract (resveratrol), green tea, neem, and ginger.

- Immune stimulants include appropriate rasayanas (amalaki, amrit, guduchi, chyavanprash, brahma rasayana, amruthaprasham). A good Ayurvedic physician or consultant can guide you in using these.

• Guided imagery, visualization, and emotional support

Manage the DNA and you manage health. Cancer is obstinate. Nevertheless, in the science-driven world of cancer treatment, Ayurveda (working at the deepest levels) has shown good results.

Removal of Ama (Impurities in the Body)[36]

Ama is a concept of Ayurveda that can be understood as accumulated toxic substances at different levels of the physiology. Leaky gut syndrome and dysbiosis contribute to the production of ama. At the level of gross digestion, poorly digested food results in a thick, slimy material that lines the walls of the bowel, impeding absorption and assimilation of nutrients. Absorption of poorly digested material and intermediate metabolites, combined with free-radical-damaged cellular material, cellular waste material, and toxins absorbed from the food supply and the environment block the channels of the physiology at different levels, leading to various diseases and disorders. This toxic material (ama) can be viewed as a foreign substance by the body and the immune system can react by forming antibodies to it, giving rise to antigen–antibody complexes and resulting in immune disorders.

At the cellular level, during functioning of the physiology, there is accumulation of impurities and toxins. These impurities come from both inside and outside the body. From inside the body come internal metabolic and cellular waste products, such as free-radical-damaged cells and tissues, and from outside come external impurities and toxins, such as herbicides, pesticides, pollutants, and toxins that occur naturally in food. All these impurities are collectively referred to as Ama.

The management of ama, in brief, begins with identifying the etiological factors—the cause. The dosha that is the root cause of ama is pacified through proper diet, daily routine, and behavior, and balancing the predominant seasonal dosha. Ama pachana (digesting ama) is done using diet, spices, and herbs. After ama pachana, oil massage is added, as well as shodhana—detoxifying or clearing ama from the physiology through following a proper diet, ingesting herbs, and undergoing panchakarma purification therapies.

Health-Promoting Herbs for Longer Life and Increased Immunity

Ayurvedic herbs and preparations known as rasayanas are another player in promoting health. We have discussed how diet influences health. When imbalances become extreme, targeted natural substances (herbs) can get the epigenetic feedback loop working to our advantage. Rasayanas are best utilized to neutralize ongoing damage to the physiology and regenerate the system. Rasayanas are most effective when the body is free of ama.

Some rasayanas that are known to be beneficial are: Maharishi Amrit Kalash, Brahma Rasayana, Ashwagandha Rasayana, Amruthaprasham Rasayana, Narasimha Rasayana, and Chyawanprash. Rasayanas have shown the following effects:

- Rejuvenation therapy by promoting vitality, stamina, and stimulating overall health

- Promotion of longevity by delay of aging process

- Increased resistance to disease

- Activation of tissue repair mechanisms

- Enhanced immunity

- Cancer prevention

- Reduced chemotherapy and radiation toxicity[55]

- Inhibition of LDL oxidation

- Reduction of severity of atherosclerosis

- Prevention of platelet aggregation

- Immunostimulatory, myeloprotective, and antioxidant effects (from Brahma Rasayana, Maharishi Amrit Kalash, and Amruthaprasham)

Super Herb: A Full-Spectrum Antioxidant

Here are some tested results for a popular herbal preparation from Maharishi Ayurveda called Maharishi Amrit Kalash (MAK). For details, see *Ayurvedic Healing* by Sharma and Clark.[36] Makes you want to get onto a regular regimen of it:

- Free radical scavenging effects

- Increased immunity

- Cancer prevention and management
     (breast, lung, neuroblastoma, melanoma, liver)

- Reduction of chemotherapy toxicity
     (adriamycin, cisplatin, clinical)

- Management of atherosclerosis
     Reduced platelet aggregation
     Reduced lipid oxidation
     Reduced atheroma

- Anti-aging effects

- Blocking of exogenous opioid receptors: MAK blocks the receptors in the brain for exogenous opioid compounds, but does not block the receptors for endogenously produced opioid peptides. This suggests MAK may be useful for the management of substance abuse.

The Benefits of Turmeric

All you have to do is add turmeric to your food when you cook. The body does the balancing and processing to restore harmony with nature. Here are some of the effects of this everyday spice.[54,60]

- Anticancer properties because it protects against DNA damage; DNA damage leads to confused cells that can become cancer cells.

- Stimulates detoxifying enzymes. Ridding the body of toxins protects against damage to the brain of the cell and hence protects against cancer.

- Anti-mutagenic and anti-tumor effects. Actually helps correct cancerous growth once they begin.

- Anti-inflammatory: To get technical for a moment, turmeric inhibits enzymes, hormones, and other biochemicals that cause inflammation (lipoxygenase, thromboxane, cyclooxygenase-2, leukotrienes, interleukin-12, hyaluronidase).

- Antioxidant, which means that it cuts down those known, cancer-causing marauders – free radicals.

- Protective of that delicate, powerful organ, the liver (hepatoprotective)

- Antibacterial and antifungal

- Promotes wound healing

- Decreases LDL and triglycerides, associated with cholesterol and heart disease. Is actually protective against blood clots (anti-thrombotic)

- Prevents lipid peroxidation and aortic streak formation, which causes blood vessel disease

- Protects cells from β-amyloid injury—may protect against Alzheimer's disease; Prevents memory deficits in an animal model (curcumin)

Such a list is quite an array of benefits from an orange powder that does not even have any aroma to speak of. Any one of the benefits makes turmeric worthwhile. Getting the entire list, as you do when you eat it, makes the herb almost impossible to pass over. It's more effective to use the whole herb than just the extract. The active ingredient, curcumin, has poor bioavailability due to poor absorption, rapid metabolism, and rapid elimination.[61] Research has also shown that other ingredients in turmeric have anti-cancer properties. A curcumin-free extract of turmeric suppresses tumors in mice and rats, slows the growth of colon cancer cells, and fights pancreatic cancer cells.[60]

The Tools of Ayurveda

Here is a list of Ayurvedic approaches to living,[53] each of which, done properly, attunes us to the deeper levels of life, and hence spurs that much-sought-after kundalini.

- *Diet and Digestion:* Ayurveda maintains that all approaches to health can be maximally effective only if appropriate dietary measures are instituted simultaneously to support the restoration of physiological balance. Ayurveda has no single diet that is purported to be suitable for all individuals and all situations. The prescription of diet is individualized, based on the diagnosis of the individual's current dosha status and taking into account seasonal influences, the individual's age and digestive capacity, any disease or imbalance present, sources and purity of food, and other factors. The optimal diet is one that tends to restore the individual to a state of balance. Digestion is of prime importance in maintaining health. The end product of truly healthy diet and digestion is said to produce significant amounts of Ojas (see below).

- *Herbs and Rasayanas:* Ayurvedic pharmacology (known as Dravyaguna) utilizes the synergistic cooperation of substances as they coexist in natural sources. It uses single plants, or more often, mixtures of plants whose effects are complementary. In terms of Ayurveda, the effectiveness of herbal mixtures may ultimately be explained by the idea that plants, especially herbs, are concentrated repositories of nature's intelligence which, when used properly, can increase the expression of that intelligence in the body. Special preparations known as rasayanas promote longevity, stamina, immunity, and overall well-being. Common spices used in cooking also have therapeutic properties.

- *Daily and seasonal routines:* Daily routine includes getting up with the sunrise, evacuating bowels and bladder, brushing teeth and scraping tongue, taking a shower, doing yoga, breathing exercises, meditation, and then eating breakfast before going to work or school. Lunch should be the main meal of the day. In the evening, eat a light dinner and then pursue a pleasant, relaxing activity, and go to bed by 10:00 p.m.

- *Changes in the season create fundamental shifts in our biochemistry and metabolic style.* Seasonal routine varies according to the predominant dosha of the season. For example, kapha accumulates in the springtime. Since this dosha is associated with the quality of heaviness, physical exercise is suggested and daytime sleep should be avoided. In summer pitta accumulates. This dosha is associated with the quality of heat, so exposure to the sun should be avoided, physical overexertion should be avoided, and light clothing should be worn. In winter, vata accumulates. This dosha is associated with qualities of coldness and dryness, so the recommendations include oil massage, exposure to the sun, and heavy, warm clothing.

- *Behavioral Rasayana and Emotions:* Behavior, speech, and emotions are important aspects of the human psyche that affect health in a dramatic way. Ayurveda includes detailed discussions of lifestyle and behavior and their impact on health. Interestingly, traditional virtues such as respect for elders, teachers, loved ones, and family members; pardoning those who wrong you; practicing nonviolence; not speaking ill of others behind their back and so on, are understood to promote health for the individual's mind and body, as well as for the community and society as a whole. The input from the five senses—hearing, sight, touch, taste, and smell creates changes in the physiology, and each experience is metabolized in its own way. Information from the different senses is metabolized and affects our behavior. Therefore, it is important to experience health-promoting input through each of the five senses. According to Ayurveda one should avoid overuse of the senses, no use of the senses, and improper use of the senses; this balance in sensory input helps maintain balance in the physiology. Emotions can be understood as fine fluctuations of consciousness; as such, their impact on the more expressed physical levels of the body is understood to be immense. Ayurveda has various modalities to keep the emotions balanced; meditation and pranayama (breathing exercises) are two of the major ones. Meditation keeps us in touch with the source of our existence, which has a balancing effect on all aspects of our Being. Pranayama activates prana, the vital energy in the body, thus balancing the body's energy field and the emotions.

- *Ojas enhancement:* Ojas is said to be the most important bio-chemical substance mediating the influence of consciousness on the body. When present in abundance, ojas gives strength, immunity, contentment, and good digestion. Inefficient digestion and metabolism, on the other hand, result in production of toxic material in the body called *Ama*, the buildup of which results in disease.

- *Purification therapies called panchakarma:* Ayurveda recommends purification therapy at the change of seasons due to the accumulation of doshas that occurs at that time. This therapy is known as panchakarma and it rids the body of toxins to prevent the onset of disease. Various modifications of this procedure are in vogue today. Traditionally, panchakarma includes two preliminary practices that begin the toxin removal process, five main techniques that complete toxin removal from the body, and follow-up practices for rejuvenation and maintenance of the benefits provided by Panchakarma. The two preliminary practices are snehana and swedana. Snehana involves external and internal oleation of the body, and swedana is heat therapy. There are five main techniques and additional therapies are also available. The modalities utilized depend on the constitution of the patient and any disturbances in the physiology. Panchakarma also includes specialized procedures for various disorders.

- *Yoga asanas:* Yoga asanas are physical postures that help remove physical stresses in the body, promote flexibility in the system, are beneficial for the internal organs, help open the nadis, the channels through which energy flows in the body, and prepare the body for meditation.

- *Pranayama* (breathing exercises)

- *Chakra balancing and activation*

- *Marma therapy:* Marma therapy involves accessing marma points on the physical body for proper flow of prana through the nadis and chakras.

- *Meditation:* This keeps us in touch with the source of our existence, which has a balancing effect on all aspects of our life.

- *Sound therapy*

- *Architectural approach to health*—Vastu

- *Collective health:* This involves programs regarding infectious diseases, epidemics, chronic diseases, and social disorders.

The list could go on and on. You don't just grab them and start doing them and expect to become a walking mass of pure energy. Ayurveda is a personalized system of health care. For best results, consult with an Ayurvedic practitioner. Go to experts with proven track records.

A Healthy Technique We All Can Relate to—Sleep

How does sleep line us up with the universe? During activity, the mind is too active for us to be connecting a lot with the universal consciousness. In sleep, all kinds of intermediary levels of human consciousness go silent—the mind, intellect, ego, and that gigantic storehouse of impressions—chitta. When they're quiet, what's left, the energy sheath, can nestle into the universal level and rejuvenate us. Sleep is absolutely a requirement for good health and an ideal example of one at that. Get your energy body lined up. We're not used to saying about sleep, "I'm heading off to bed to get my energy body lined up. I'm shutting down my overactive chitta. I need this. I'll be a better person." But lining up is exactly what we're doing.

Sleep, we all know, is important. By one reliable estimate, lack of sleep causes $411 billion a year in lost productivity in the US workforce according to a study by the nonprofit RAND corporation in Santa Monica, CA.[62] We know people are wandering around offices and factories like zombies and getting paid for it. Lack of sleep costs us money.

A lack of sleep causes the buildup of ama, a toxic substance that clogs the nadis.

But good chemicals in our body known as cytokines build up in response to fatigue and toxins. Get some sleep, and those cytokines can thrive and help cell communication, which increases our health in all kinds of ways. The cytokine TNF (tumor necrosis factor) that scavenges cancer cells increases by tenfold during sleep. Sleep is anti-cancer therapy. Another cytokine that increases is interferon, which has anti-viral properties.

Another cytokine, Interleukin-2, a potent anticancer chemical, gets a chance during sleep to increase. Melatonin, a hormone that helps initiate sleep, also increases during sleep.

The hormone prolactin, mainly known as the protein to help women produce milk after childbirth, is also important to both male and female reproductive health. It is secreted in deep sleep, and this helps white blood cell activity which is a component of the immune system. For more details, see *The Answer to Cancer* by Sharma, et al.[14] Sleep. Simple sleep. It's a health-promoting technique of the highest order. If you want to give your vata, pitta, and kapha a chance to communicate with their source in pure consciousness, go to bed early and keep regular sleeping hours.

Other Important Basic Practices

Kundalini. Chakras. Swirling masses of energy. This sounds like a wonderful thing to have as part of our lives. Meanwhile, we go slogging through life working too hard, eating convenience foods on the fly, staying up late to watch Jimmy Kimmel, and going to the doctor now and then for prescriptions when we don't feel well.

Chakras sound great. But how in the world do we wake them up? How in the world do we move up from the bottom one, which has to do with animal instincts, to something higher that has to do with, say, the third eye and liberation? One thing seems clear. There are incentives for doing something to make us move into the higher chakras. If beneficial changes happen in the energy system, they show up later in the physiological system. We can go from feeling sick to feeling healthy, or even feeling better than that by engaging in life-changing routines.

Physical Postures—Yoga Asanas

Yoga, back before the millennials came of age, was an essentially lost and buried practice. No one contorted the body into uncomfortable positions and held them for a long time. Then a few yoga studios were established in Greenwich Village and upscale parts of LA, and the word spread that yoga asanas were very good for you. Soon it seemed like everybody was doing them.

The asanas do not in themselves cause the mind to move beyond the physical level to those deep, transcendental levels that are beyond the DNA. They can be soothing and stabilizing, though as they get rid of some of the physical stresses in the body and are beneficial to the internal organs. And they're an excellent preparation for going deep inside in meditation.

Pranayama—Breathing Exercises

Pranayama includes various types of breathing exercises that balance and increase prana. Pranayama balances both sides of the brain and balances the emotions. It opens up the nadis. Like the yoga asanas, pranayama is excellent for stabilizing the system before going within in meditation.

Meditation

Like yoga, meditation has become an everyday word and an everyday practice. If, during meditation such as Transcendental Meditation or other Vedic practices, the mind goes beyond the gross physical level to those deep, inner energy levels, the flow of kundalini in the body increases. A combination of a few yoga asanas followed by a few minutes of pranayama and twenty minutes of deep meditation opens up the flow of kundalini in the body and, hence, enlivens the DNA.

Primordial Sound Therapy

Certain sounds, such as chanting of portions of the Veda, resonate with the systems in the body that are the expression of those sounds. Listening to appropriate sound therapy can cause our body to resonate to these sounds and help it return to its healthy and balanced base condition, and thereby open channels for kundalini.

If all this is new to you, it can seem like a bombardment of information. You might think, "Wait a second. Okay, I should do some yoga positions. But which ones? I know herbal supplements can probably help me. But how do I know my body type so I get the right ones? Turmeric is said to be really good for you. But it doesn't have much taste, and I don't cook with it. What would taste good with turmeric? Telling me to get enough sleep is easy for you to say. And I don't understand how gems are good for you or all this stuff about sound therapy."

If you work with an Ayurvedic consultant, the recommendations can become quite manageable and something you can incorporate readily. It will become clear to you that you are just learning to attune your phenotype (your body) to the universe.

If you're looking for one simple, powerful way to attune to the universe, you may find that meditation is the right way. You can do it. It is the most basic, universal Ayurvedic practice for diving beyond the physical level into the energy levels and into pure consciousness itself.

15

Meditation:
A Maha Kundalini Booster

OK. The fusillade of alternative techniques can seem overwhelming. "I just want to balance my chakras," one can say. "I'm not a doctor. I'm not a yoga instructor. I'm certainly not a food faddist. I'm probably not going to move to a different house. And stress comes to me uninvited." The one powerful technique for bringing life force to the body, increasing ojas, and avoiding disease is meditation. Close the eyes, and the kundalini rises and travels throughout the body.

Why Meditation is So Promising

Epigenetics brings hope. Thanks to the feedback loop, when DNA expresses itself, we can turn genes on and off and move them in the right direction. Thinking of the same process in terms of vata, pitta, kapha, and sattva, rajas, and tamas, we can enliven ojas in the system, which means that we balance those three doshas. When they're balanced, they reflect the universe, which is all powerful.

The litany of meditation types can leave us in a quandary about choices. There's the meditation people learn to do after yoga class. There are audio tapes of guided meditations. There's Christian meditation, much akin to prayer. There's Buddhist meditation. There's chanting. Often we're looking for the same result from the practice of meditation–to find peace by experiencing our essential nature in attunement with the universe.

Different Meditations and Different Brain Waves

Whenever we can turn to science for validation and understanding, we have a solid, repeatable basis for our conclusions. One study, for example, categorizes meditations in three ways: Focused Attention, Open Monitoring, and Automatic Self-Transcending.[63]

1. Focused-Attention Meditation

- Examples of this are Tibetan Buddhist "loving kindness and compassion," Zen and the Diamond Way Buddhist technique, and Chinese Qigong meditation.

- Beta/Gamma activity in brain—Gamma waves associated with highly active brain.

- These types of meditation do not support experiences of quieter levels of the mind, nor the peace and silence of Yoga; i.e., they don't open up the gateways to kundalini.

2. Open Monitoring (Mindfulness-based Meditation)

- Non-reactive monitoring of the content of ongoing experience.

- Being cognizant of thought or breath, e.g., Buddhist Mindfulness, ZaZen, Chinese Qigong, and Sahaj Yoga meditation.

- Increased frontal midline theta and increased occipital gamma power—associated with more active brain.

- These types of meditation do not bring the experience of Yoga.

3. Automatic Self-Transcending (Transcendental Meditation, some Vedic technologies)

- No concentration or focus.

- Global coherent Alpha waves—associated with experience of peace, the state of Yoga.

- Decreased beta1 and gamma power.

- Neural imaging—increased blood flow to prefrontal cortex and decreased blood flow to thalamus and basal ganglia indicates a state of restful alertness.

- Supports experience of deep rest and increased alertness during meditation.

Focused attention: This may be the type of meditation the person on the street thinks of when he/she says, "I've tried it. I just can't do it." People think the objective is to clear the mind of thoughts in order to concentrate on something, and for some types of meditation that is the objective. With focused attention the beta/gamma activity increases, which correlates with a high level of activity in the brain. With these types of meditation the mind does not experience quieter levels (which is where the energy body takes up residence).

Open monitoring: This is being relaxed and aware of your thoughts or your breathing. (At least with this we don't face the challenge of trying to stop our thoughts altogether.) Many forms of mindfulness meditation fall into this category. The purpose is to be in the present moment. What kind of brain waves do we get? Theta and gamma. These techniques are popular and they have a following. You can learn them for free. You can pick them up on the Internet and even begin teaching them. Psychologists love them as a way to help people relax. These meditations do not give the experience of Yoga (also called Samadhi, which means union with those silent inner energy fields we've been mentioning).

Automatic self-transcending: If the name describes what is happening, then this meditation does get us below the threshold of the DNA and into the energy body, the field of kundalini. Transcendental Meditation and other Vedic meditations accomplish it. These techniques do not involve concentration. The waves are increased frontal alpha and decreased beta1 and gamma power, and increased frontal alpha1 coherence. And—big relief—alpha does associate with the state of Yoga, the experience of inner peace and inner union with those fields beneath the surface of life. Finally, a dive. The imaging studies suggest a state of restful alertness. Rest and alertness at the same time. An apparent paradox, but the brain loves it and begins pumping kundalini.

With practices like Transcendental Meditation where the mind goes below the surface, the mind actually becomes one with that amazingly powerful cosmic prana (which becomes all-transforming kundalini in the cells of the body). In the epigenetics feedback loop, that rising kundalini is the instrument for turning on helpful genes and turning off damaging ones.

Brain Wave Frequencies and How They Affect Us and Make Us Feel

We're not in the habit of looking at our brain wave frequencies. But a lot is at stake during meditation, namely getting into the energy body and beyond into pure consciousness. The brain waves resulting from each kind of meditation—gamma for concentration techniques, theta for monitoring inner processes and mental imagery, and alpha for deep relaxation affect us differently. The other brain waves involved are beta, which go with our normal waking state, and delta waves that we experience during deep sleep.

Here are the different ways our brain waves affect us:

Gamma waves, 40–100 Hz

Associated with intense focus and concentration

Too many cause anxiety and stress

Too few can cause ADHD and depression

Beta waves, 12–40 Hz

Exist in a waking state—processing of information

Too many cause anxiety and inability to relax

Too few causes ADHD and depression

Increased by coffee, energy drinks, and stimulants

Alpha waves, 8–12 Hz

Are the bridge between conscious and subconscious

Cause deep relaxation

Too few cause stress and anxiety

Theta waves, 4–8 Hz

Monitor inner processes and mental imagery

Exist during daydreaming and sleep

Experienced when feeling deep and raw emotions

Too many cause ADHD, depression, and inattentiveness

Delta waves, 0.5–4 Hz

Are associated with stage N3 slow-wave sleep, which is deep sleep

Study Showing TM Flips on and off the Right Genes

John Fagan, PhD, from the Maharishi University of Management, has presented research on the effect of self-transcending meditation on gene expression.[13] This study on the Transcendental Meditation (TM) technique found that TM decreased the expression of 56 genes and increased that of 18 genes, compared to healthy controls matched by age, sex, diet, and tobacco and alcohol use that did not do the TM technique. What did those genes do? The scientists say, in summary, that genes involved in the stress response, inflammation, and cardiovascular disease were generally found to be reduced in expression. Two tumor suppressor genes were found to be increased in expression. Stress, we know, is the dreaded kundalini blocker. Inflammation is a predecessor to many degenerative diseases. And of course we want our tumor suppressor genes to be active.

What we're looking for with all this cavalcade of New Age techniques, from gems to yoga postures to spices, is to find a way to cross the threshold from the everyday level into the magic kingdom of those inner energy fields. Automatic self-transcending may be a leading candidate for doing that.

Telomeres and Neuroplasticity

As we mentioned previously, a large number of research studies have been published on the effects of meditation. Here are a few known, scientifically tested results of meditation practices.[12,64,65]

- Meditation repairs genetic expression of illness, e.g., prostate cancer

- Extends life of cells by preventing shortening of telomeres

- Improves brain functioning by synchronizing functions of both sides of brain

- Improves neuroplasticity by changing neural pathways and synapses, resulting in healthy development, learning, and memory

- GABA activity increases, which keeps negativity under control

Do you have a favorite from the list? "Prevents shortening of telomeres" is enticing. Telomeres shorten as we age. If we prevent the shortening, we live longer. "Neuroplasticity" sounds good, too, which can mean improved or at least maintained memory. If we're going to have longer telomeres and thereby live into old age, we'd hate to run smack into memory loss along the way.

I think my personal favorite from the list is "GABA activity increases." GABA is actually gamma-aminobutyric acid. It's Valium. Not literally. But it is a tranquilizer, a natural tranquilizer. Sometimes it seems like we could take all the rest of the discussion around epigenetics and happiness and beating aging and just settle in with a nice tranquilizer. Well, here it is. GABA from meditation. That's all we need to know.

Here is another summary of scientifically verified effects of meditation.[66]

Scientifically Verified Benefits of Meditation

- Feeling more peaceful

- Increase in ability to get over anxiety and grief

- Increase in ability to overcome pain, physical or psychological

- Improvement of health

- Increase in ability to break negative habit patterns

- Increase in ability to be sensitive, intuitive, and discerning

- Improvement of memory

- More fulfilling relationships

- Increase of mental power and improvement of efficiency

So meditation is a pain reliever. Does "Ability to break negative habit patterns" mean, like, recovery from addiction? It does, actually. Effective meditation with transcending is quite helpful in treating addiction. Serotonin grows in the system as a result of meditation, and it's fulfilling.[67] (For those just looking to get high, read on, because kundalini can be a real buzz, man.)

Scientific Articles on Meditation

Scientific research changes the ball game from guesswork, baseless hoping, mood-making, and superstition into valid, credible results. The results do seem to lean rather heavily toward one approach, Transcendental Meditation (TM). TM pioneered in scientific research for a field that once was thought to be purely spiritual and subjective and, hence, not available for testing. There are many references, for those who are interested.[15,51,68–77] The point is that there is scientific research on meditation techniques for improving health, and therefore, by extension, using the epigenetic feedback loop to flip the right genes on and the wrong ones off.

One Maha Kundalini Booster

With so many ways to perk up kundalini, what we really need is one powerful candidate with some kind of a central organizing principle, such as the increasing of inner consciousness. Yoga and pranayama help take us in the direction of those inner energy fields and consciousness fields that are the true kundalini boosters. If the meditation accomplishes that, the others, done in the right way and sometimes with supervision, can enhance it. But some basic dive-into-the-Absolute practice can be the foundation for everything else.

We need the right thing to get us rolling with our quest for more kundalini. However we do it, we want to get that feedback loop really cranking so that a lot of good things can happen—even the best things of all—perfect health, supernormal abilities, and whatever is our highest possibility in the universe. Let's do more than lowering our blood pressure a little and not getting too overweight.

Part Four

The Light Body

16

Just Having Good Health Is a Gyp

The subject of health, excuse me, is generally just boring. Who cares about it except when it goes downhill? Most people, most of the time, are not dying from some dreaded disease. Therefore, in the parlance of the modern world, they're healthy. Maybe they're dragging themselves around tired. Maybe they fly off the handle at the least incident and continue to flutter for an hour or two afterward. Maybe they can't sleep. Maybe they overeat. That is what we call "normal" and "healthy." When you have to call in hospice help, I suppose then you're really sick. I had a friend with cancer (he later died from it) who was paralyzed from the waist down. He kept working. He felt pretty good. He described himself as "the healthiest dying man the docs have ever seen."

We have to aim for more than generally good health when we elevate the DNA, and, lo and behold, we do just that. When you look at some of the capabilities Ayurveda talks about in our swirling energy systems throughout the body, not getting colds or being able to sleep well at night seem like just the beginning of what we can enjoy by purifying our system and strengthening the DNA. Why would we settle for having just those simple things?

Kundalini Shakti—Primal Energy Flowing Freely

Having kundalini shakti ("shakti" means "power") should be our goal. This is the flow of unobstructed primal energy throughout the body. Doesn't that sound like something worth having? Here in quick summary are the effects of kundalini shakti in each chakra:

Kundalini Really Lights You Up

- When passing through sushumna (one of the three main nadis) all nadis, chakras, and the entire body emanates that shakti.

- When passing through mooladhara chakra (the root chakra) the sense of smell becomes acute, intuitive knowledge increases, writing ability develops, natural ecstasy occurs.

- When passing through swadhisthana chakra (the sacral chakra) the sense of taste becomes very sharp. There is no fear of water, a psychic ability and control of senses develops, and perception of the astral realm and intuition become heightened.

- When passing through manipura chakra (the navel chakra) the body is free of disease; excretions, hunger, and thirst decrease, excess fat is lost, and skin becomes radiant.

- When passing through anahat chakra (the heart chakra) this arouses inner sounds or nada; pranic healing becomes apparent; the individual becomes sensitive toward others and external vibrations; immense compassion and love for all beings arises.

- Passing through vishuddhi chakra (the throat chakra) the voice becomes melodious and resonant and words become totally captivating.

- When kundalini reaches ajna chakra (the third eye chakra) pure knowledge and wisdom unfold.

- When kundalini reaches sahasrara chakra (crown chakra) perfection is attained.

It is well worth relishing the benefits of the full flow of kundalini in each chakra, so let's do that. I think even just reading about the benefits tends to enliven them a little bit.

Writing Ability of Chaucer and Shakespeare

It shouldn't be totally surprising that when kundalini shakti passes through the lowest chakra (mooladhara chakra), writing ability develops. Writers throughout the ages have brought the base levels of life to the surface to the delight of readers. Geoffrey Chaucer in England of the Middle Ages played at length with those lowest levels in hilarious comedies like "The Miller's Tale." Countryman William Shakespeare centuries later could create the most ribald and brutish of scenes when called upon. Writing is not all that flourishes from that lowest chakra. How about natural ecstasy? People risk prison, serious addictions, loss of other faculties, and general confusion for even brief bouts of ecstasy from various opiates and barbiturates, one of which is even named "Ecstasy." What is it worth to get all that naturally?

Psychic Ability

Moving to the next chakra, only slightly further up the spine, kundalini awakens another world of delights. Sense of taste becomes very sharp, for example. Many a gourmand has known the joys of savory vegetable biryani concoctions heightened with coriander chutney. What a satisfaction to have that chakra open—with so much more to delight in than an everyday feeling of "being well."

Psychic ability develops. Wrongly associated only with the highest chakra, psychic ability actually resides here in the loins, delighting and surprising a person and his/her friends as the person reveals the past or predicts the future, or knows what you are thinking before you say it.

Control of the senses grows, and the ability to refrain from excesses is useful for someone living an indulgent existence. Perception of the astral realm increases as swadhisthana opens. A great companion to psychic ability, perception of the astral realm is also a popular way to impress your incredulous friends. Intuition flourishes.

If all this comes from kundalini flow in the lowest of chakras, what wonders await us as we move up the spine? Are there any super powers left?

Third Chakra and No Disease?

The next chakra up the chain, manipura chakra, relates to health and freedom from disease. Get the kundalini surging through it, and you might have a disease-free body. Meanwhile, your body operates so efficiently that excretions decrease. Being so efficient in digestion and the operation of your circulation, your hunger decreases. You'll have appeal from your good health and balance. Your skin becomes radiant. That alone makes a person attractive.

Love for Lizards, Snakes, Clouds, People, Everything

We can expect a lot from a chakra associated with the heart, and we are not to be disappointed. Moving beyond freedom from disease at the previous chakra, at the anahat chakra we begin to experience pranic healing—powerful healing at the first, bubbling, nearly all-powerful level of creation. We grow in the right kind of sensitivity to others, which they universally appreciate. Compassion blossoms, and we feel love not just for fellow humans but for chipmunks, spiders, lions, palm trees, and every other form of being. We dissolve in love. Could anything be better than that?

Beyond Sinatra—Operatic.

Singing is one of the highest undertakings. Even your everyday rock singer can be mesmerizing. As this chakra experiences the flow of kundalini, the voice becomes truly strong—resonant and melodious. In some famous stories of enlightenment, everyone realizes what has happened when they hear the sweet sounds through the forest from the newly enlightened soul. He melts in the joy of his own expression while delighting all the creatures around him. Should such a man or woman speak, everyone is not just fascinated, but totally captivated. They hang on his/her every word. Such a person can influence millions.

Pure Knowledge

With so much gained from lower chakras, what more can we expect from a higher one, such as the Ajna chakra, perched at the top of the spinal column? Pure knowledge and wisdom unfolds. One becomes all-knowing. If there is anything one might ask for, such as success in business or improvement in family relations, you know exactly how to get it. Knowledge is power. This, being pure knowledge, is pure power.

Are you omniscient? Do you know everything everywhere in the universe all the time? No. But you have all knowledge about anything, in a single point. Whatever you need, you know. And you have a comfortable sense of all-knowingness inside.

Perfection

With so much gained already from the lower six chakras, what more could possibly come from the highest? Dream of dreams. Here there is nothing piecemeal. Whatever you might want from the previous levels—writing ability, a great singing voice, fine culinary abilities—whatever you want—you get it all. You gain, if we can be so bold, perfection. You are still human. You are not the creator. But you are a perfected human.

Mere health, then? In the world we found ourselves wandering through, health sounded like enough to ask for. People had weight problems. Their livers made them cross and fidgety. They couldn't focus. They had a sore shoulder or foot or chronic back problem. Sometimes it seems like enough just to have some relief. Decent health seems like a worthy target. But only until you attain it. Then you want something more.

If our best systems just get us to the point where we are functional without a lot of issues, what have they done for us truly? More, more, more. Once we get some stability, we don't just remain stationary. Nature is a force of evolution. It pushes us forward, toward more and more. Psychic abilities. Refined taste. Pure knowledge. Knowledge of almost everything. Perfect the DNA and gain all those abilities. That's something worth doing.

17

Past Lives and Future Lives

If kundalini, operating through the DNA, can propel us into powers, can it protect us from diseases and tragedies that we are now carrying in our DNA? Can it protect us not just from what we bring with us from our parents, but what we bring from their parents, and theirs? Can it protect us from what we've brought with us from our own past lives and what we might otherwise have to face in our future lives? For those who are skeptics about past and future lives, reincarnation, and near-death experiences, there are well-documented cases that have been described in publications authored by Western medicine physicians, researchers, and others.[78–93]

The Curse of the Kennedys

There's even a name for karma that carries over through generations. A family known for living in "Camelot" and sometimes called the First Family of America, has faced tragedy across generations. Joseph P. Kennedy, Jr. died in a plane crash in WW II. President John F. Kennedy was assassinated, and his brother Robert likewise was killed while campaigning for President. Edward Kennedy, Jr., had bone cancer and a leg amputation when he was twelve. Michael Kennedy died in a skiing accident when he went headfirst into a tree. John F. Kennedy, Jr., broke the hearts of a nation and the world when he died at the age of thirty-eight in a plane crash. A book, *The Sins of the Father: Joseph P. Kennedy and the Dynasty He Founded*[94] actually says in print what many people cannot help suspecting—that somehow misbehaviors in the past have been passed on to children and grandchildren in the present, and will continue to be.

The tragedy in itself is of course monumental, but it stands in stark contrast to the wealth, the grandeur, the power, the charisma. Yes, John F. Kennedy became president, like Dwight D. Eisenhower before him and Lyndon Baines Johnson afterward. But JFK was a heartthrob, a movie star on the world stage, a paragon of sheer, dashing, compelling intelligence and power and eloquence.

In Greek tragedies like the story of Agamemnon, the king first commits an egregious wrong, killing his daughter to appease the gods. Later, his wife Clytemnestra kills him, and the action and reaction seem like the clear working of karma.

You don't have to be a Kennedy or a Greek mythic figure to have family karma. Cancer runs in families. Heart disease afflicts some families more than others. Diabetes troubles Native American families more than others, and sickle cell anemia plagues African Americans.

It's in the DNA

What is now coming to the forefront is that family curses reside in the DNA. Scientists now know that DNA gets damaged by stress.[95–97] That damaged DNA is transferred to the progeny. Diseases are hereditary.

Actions make impressions, even small actions, let alone grand actions like Agamemnon putting his daughter to the sword. Negative actions like sneaking into the movie theater and speaking ill of your best friend behind his/her back are imprinted. So are positive actions, such as striking up a friendly conversation with your neighbor or giving a chew toy to a puppy. You're recording everything in your DNA.

It's amazing how sensitive the DNA is. DNA is linked with the pranic body which, sitting next to the unmanifest level, is totally sensitive and powerful. For instance, in the laboratory, researchers have taken a tube and emptied it out. Distribution of photons in the tube was random. When they placed DNA in the tube, the distribution became orderly and remained so even after they removed the DNA.[98]

Take a swab of DNA from a person, put it in a tube in the next room, and then create different emotions in the person. Make him happy. Startle him. Make him sad. The DNA in the tube changes. It reacts to what the man feels. Emotions affect the DNA. Move the DNA 50 miles away and the DNA reacts just as much, and does so instantaneously.[99] Introduce positive emotions, and the DNA in the tube unwinds and can express itself. Introduce negative emotions, and it contracts and cannot express itself.[100,101]

Children have DNA from both parents and not only carry the emotions in the DNA from the time of conception, but continue to respond to emotions of the parents throughout life. If something happens to a child, sometimes the mother knows instantly.

Not Just the Parents But Theirs and Theirs and Theirs

The DNA doesn't just carry information from the current parents. Those parents, after all, contain DNA from their parents, and so on and so on and so on. That delicate film of the DNA is so sensitive that it doesn't forget anything, even from decades before. You don't have to go very far back to get to times when lives were short and behaviors were harsh. Fathers routinely hit their children and carried the memory of that in their DNA.

Whole nations and ethnic groups carry both the shining glories of their pasts and the dark stresses as well. Take a nation like Jamaica, peopled by captured slaves. Fear has continued as a way of life, along with strength, perseverance, and athleticism. Jews are not about to forget the Holocaust, and even if they should forget it consciously, the DNA does not forget. How about Cambodians who lived through the Pol Pot genocide of the late seventies? It sits in the DNA. Of course, it's not just trauma that affects the DNA. Positive attributes are carried across generations as well. For example, Native Americans, in some instances, make excellent skyscraper workers because they do not fear heights.

You Carry the Actions of Your Own Previous Lives

"There. I'll die soon. That should take care of everything." That's what we tend to think. Death is final. It wipes out everything. "You can't take it with you." But you should never underestimate the effects of your actions. They don't get wiped out with the body. Like the gopher in Bill Murray's *Caddyshack* scenes, they refuse to go away, no matter what you do.

It's one thing to think of your DNA reflecting the past behaviors of your grandmother or hers or hers. This is something else. It reflects past behaviors of your own in previous lives. Your past impressions don't die when the body dies. They remain in the subtle body.

Take this a step further. They remain in seed form to come back to you in your future incarnations. Those tender inner energy fields, known to Ayurveda, are there in all their rich recording. The totality of you. All those aspects we discussed previously. As a reminder, here they are again, this time with their functions listed too. Here is the Ayurvedic view of you, me, and any individual:

- Physical Body

    Physical Sheath—Life and death

    Energy Sheath (Life force)—Energy, hunger and thirst

- Inner Faculty (Working Consciousness)

    Mind—Sensory processing, duality—likes and dislikes, happiness and sadness

Intellect—Deciding, discriminating, judging (lack of correct perspective, or mistake of the intellect)

Chitta—Mind-stuff, storehouse of memories, impressions of actions are embedded here

Ego—Self sense of experiencer and doer

- Inner Being—Self

Witness, Truth, Consciousness, Indivisible, Non-dual, Peace, Bliss, Home of all the laws of Nature

Can You Fix a Curse?

Can we fix the tragic aspect of the past with diet? For example, if someone with a pitta/kapha body type spent his/her life getting attuned to nature with the right foods, would that provide protection against tragedy?

How about minimizing stress? If we did yoga asanas, pranayama, and meditation, would that create the conditions in our DNA to protect us from an oncoming disease or health problem? What about our environment? Should we live in homes with the rooms oriented properly in the right direction for us? Should we avoid using south entrances, where the most negative influences come in?

What about lifestyle and behaviors? Suppose we followed the guidelines of the Behavioral Rasayanas: Transcend on a regular basis. Speak truthfully, but sweetly. Speak well of others. Never spread gossip. Be free of anger. Abstain from alcohol and immoderate behavior. Be nonviolent and calm. Would that protect us from tragedy? How? Would it protect our children from tragedy? Would it protect us when we are reborn in another body?

Yes, You Can Reverse a Curse.

We change our karma all the time. The more we build in the positive influences of lifestyle, managing stress, following a nourishing and uplifting diet, and minimizing environmental stress, the more we enjoy health, longevity, happiness, and peace. Epigenetics means that we can modify the effects of past actions, for ourselves and for our descendants. It's not guesswork and metaphysics and theology anymore. It's physical, anchored by the DNA.

But how far can we go in raising ourselves up?

18

Perfection? Why Not? Nature Is Perfect.

When people live the right lifestyle, eat right, and manage their stress, the feedback loop causes the DNA to open up. Then the DNA sends messages to create better and better conditions in the cells. The more the cells are functioning well, the more they express inner energy fields and even pure consciousness. If we rejuvenate the cells, the sky is the limit. If we do not, how can we expect high performance from them? There is so much to be gained from clearing all the nadis. The whole system can be running like clockwork.

Well-Running Feedback Loop

As we've explained, the body has its feedback loop: from DNA to RNA to protein and then back to DNA. Suppose you had a loop in a car engine. You clean the spark plugs, clean the carburetor so you in fact have everything new, and then if you get the highest quality gas, you can have a high-performance engine.

How about getting to a high-performance body? If the feedback loop keeps refining and refining and refining the DNA, why even reach any limit? We have the right lifestyle, manage our stress, have a nourishing environment, eat right, and we refine and refine and refine. For a strong basis we do yoga asanas, pranayama, and regular meditation. We enhance it all with some light-gem therapy that enlivens the chakras. "Lather. Rinse. Repeat." We keep cleansing and cleansing the self. Karma gets stronger. Disease is averted. Powers grow.

Can We Have a Perfectly Functioning Physiology?

It should be possible, suggests scientist Dr. Robert Keith Wallace, in his book *The Physiology of Consciousness*.[102] He says, "With full knowledge of the human genome from modern science and complete comprehension of the dynamics of the expression of natural law from Maharishi's Vedic Physiology, it should be possible to fully understand the fundamental principles and processes associated with the proper expression of genetic information and the mechanics of how to permanently enliven the memory of a perfectly functioning physiology."

He explains that the ideal is to have frictionless flow of the information from the DNA to every system and organ in the body. Parts of the body harmonize with the whole. The whole harmonizes with the parts. And at the basis of it all are what he calls "homeostatic feedback loops."

He says further that coherence from the DNA benefits the whole body as the person progresses through stages of development. The immune system grows strong and stays strong, with remarkable results like preventing disease, living long, and even enjoying perfect health.

Today, It's All About Fighting Disease

Today, in our health-care system we do not see a physician to check on our degree of perfection. With a stethoscope, an array of test results, and his/her trained eye, the physician looks for . . . disease.

The model of perfection in use today is primarily something like, "You are at risk. I want you to change your diet, exercise more, and take these medications." It is not "you know, we can perk up the kundalini in your liver cells a little, open up the nadis leading to your brain, tweak your digestion, and then you will be just about perfect." We never hear that.

Start at Birth; Don't Stop

With full knowledge of the body's energy systems and the techniques to balance them, we could more and more use perfection as our ideal. By knowing prakriti (body type), we could classify infants at birth. "This is a kapha baby." "This one is vata pitta." Because we know the associations of prakriti with metabolism, chronic diseases, and genotypes, we could recommend a lifetime of personalized prevention.

"This person is at risk of obesity." Ayurveda recommends a diet that favors pungent, bitter, and astringent tastes and light, dry, and warm foods. It advises reducing heavy, oily, and cold foods and sweet, sour, and salty tastes. The details can be much more specific to the individual and vary with season of the year, and even time of the day. Imagine, though, sustaining such an appropriate diet year after year after year from birth. The benefits are cumulative as the body becomes stronger, and the feedback loop opens more and more to build inner strength.

Add in the right lifestyles. "This person will be lively and creative." "This person may not learn as quickly as some, but once he learns he won't forget." Manage stress. Meditate regularly. Then good health can be commonplace.

Percolating Infinity

The regular routine for a growing child can add in more and more purifiers. Match exercise routine to body type, for example. All children exercise, but with a lifelong health regimen, the routine can be rigorous for kapha types who can sustain it and milder and pleasanter for vata types who do well with an easier routine. Follow their progress, and make modifications as needed. This happens as a lifelong experience with children, but doing so with full knowledge of body type, the feedback loop, and DNA, raises the possibility of perfection.

What a world we're looking at, where every system and every cell in the body is open to the kundalini. What would we become? We would be nothing but consciousness itself. If consciousness were flat, this would not amount to all that much. But instead it is percolating infinity, containing the seed of all knowledge and all creativity.

19

The Light Body

Powers, overcoming the weaknesses in DNA across generations, and perfection—these are worthy goals. They are certainly worthy milestones on the journey of life. DNA, though, does not stop at milestones. It is the mirror of the universe, and the universe is gargantuan. It goes for it all.

The Purpose of Life

What is the purpose of our life? Nobody knows. Few think about it. If you're sitting around a barbeque on Memorial Day weekend, you wouldn't ask, "Hey, everybody, what's the purpose of life?" Quizzical looks would happen on all sides, with people knowingly exchanging glances that say, "We always knew this guy was different."

Who thinks about the purpose of life, even in passing? Philosophers have made pronouncements about it, but—news flash!—nobody pays them any mind at all. Head in the clouds. Feet in the clouds. Purveyors of meaningless distinctions. Evaluators of mind-twisting conundrums not to be taken seriously. Aristotle of course must have had some good points about life. Some think he said things like, *"We are what we repeatedly do. Excellence is not an act, but a habit."* Others think it is a misquote, namely, what someone else thinks Aristotle should have said. Fine.

The cynical existentialists reportedly said some discouraging things. Schopenhauer is quoted as saying, "Life swings like a pendulum backward and forward between pain and boredom." Dostoevsky asserted that we're basically cockroaches anyway. So of course we wouldn't think about something as nebulous as the purpose of life.

Thoreau pointed out pithily that the masses of us lead lives of quiet desperation. In such a state, what do we think about? A little relief from somewhere. Anywhere. We don't think about the meaning of life, and, should we decide to wax philosophical, it would be something like, "Life is hard," which still begs the question of what it's for.

DNA is a relatively recent addition to the conversation, and, until even more recently, not a particularly welcome one. DNA's message was always, "I don't change. I am what I am, and that is the end of it." Now, enter epigenetics, and there's a whole new spin on things. Epigenetics is changing the tenor of the conversation from "we can't change many of the characteristics we were born with" to "we can change what we are." What does that do to the rules of the game?

Now It's Not Nebulous. It's Physical.

The one serious, hard thing about it all is that DNA is an actual substance. We know it's an actual substance. It's a chemical, and it's as real as epinephrine or carbohydrates or lymphocytes. It's real. We can see it. We can measure it. We can test it.

Now, the DNA feedback loop changes the whole game, and I don't mean the scientific research game. I mean the game of your life and my life. The feedback loop tells us that we don't have to settle. We're not stuck. We can change our most fundamental being by flipping genes on and off. And we change them basically and fundamentally by how we live.

The fact that we change our basic nature by how we live, and that the changes get recorded in an unfailing chemical (the DNA), reconfigures the whole approach we take to the purpose of life. Now, our DNA is watching. We cannot deny our own DNA. Now, all of a sudden, we can measure our progress toward a goal. With tools from Ayurveda, we can know, physically, how we are doing.

We can raise the state of our bodies and using the feedback loop, perfect the DNA. It can handle all the perfecting we can give it, because it is the shimmering web of Absolute pure consciousness made manifest. It can handle anything that the Absolute can handle, and there is nothing that the Absolute cannot handle. (The Absolute means what physics calls the unified field or, in even more advanced discussions, the superstring.)

We have seen we can raise these levels through improvement of our lifestyle including our diet and nutrition, management of stress, and proper environment, sleep habits, and daily routine. Anything that gets us reflecting those mahabhutas (or, in physics, the five spin types) that are the fundamental elements of creation as it becomes manifest. When we get ourselves more and more attuned to that infinite that is the world and has always been the world, I think the purpose of life emerges.

When the body flourishes, it doesn't have to stop with merely good health. What else begins to flourish? It's not just that the cells are in good working order. Those inner levels shine. Let us remind you of them again:

Inner Faculty (Working Consciousness)

> Mind
>
> Intellect
>
> Chitta
>
> Ego

Inner Being—Self, Witness

My favorite is chitta—the storehouse of impressions. How incredible to have that flourish. Does it mean that we can know anything? I think it does. Having the others become sharp is good, too. The more we develop the intellect, the more we have excellent intuition. Eventually we can have all knowledge in a single point.

Prana, we have said, is the life energy. I like to think of it as that percolating level where the superstring first becomes manifest, where, from this incredible energy, life first emerges from unmanifest Absolute. This amazing energy on the surface of the Absolute is still not something we can work with. When it enters the body, though, the body transforms it into force. Life force—the resonant, fundamental life force of kundalini.

As kundalini, it is in every nucleated cell in the body. Shining, pulsating, bursting with pure light and energy. It is irresistible. In Whitman's "Song of Myself" he says, "I celebrate myself, and sing myself, And what I assume you shall assume, For every atom belonging to me as good belongs to you. I loafe and invite my soul, I lean and loafe at my ease observing a spear of summer grass." As life force bursts through our hearts and veins and arteries, through our livers and pancreases and medulla oblongatas and cerebellums and thalamuses, more and more we begin to live life as it really is.

The Light Body Is the Ultimate.

If you start at the top, with say a tree or the building across the street or your body on the surface, that is the gross level of creation. The most manifest level of life is the gross level, and then it moves to subtle levels and on to subtler levels.

In the body, the direction is the opposite—from lower to higher—but the result is the same. As we live more and more in the higher chakras, and less and less in the lower ones, we live a more refined life, a more heavenly life. We say that we evolve into higher beings. Two people can both be in life as humans, but one can be a higher being and the other a lower one. Inside of us, prana connects the subjective level of our life (mind, intellect, chitta, ego) to the physical body.

Those subjective levels can be there and just be insentient. Then, as the light of consciousness falls on them, they become sentient. Here the game begins to become truly the game. To have more consciousness fall on them, we need to have more and more kundalini (life force).

When we live in this life, how we live determines how much consciousness we reflect. There really are no shortcuts other than certain forms of meditation. Whatever vibrational level we reach, that is the level we reach. If we happen to drop the body, we don't miraculously ascend to the highest heaven by virtue of having died. We stay at the same level where we are. In the afterlife, we find ourselves among people of the same vibrational level. "In my Father's house are many mansions," Christ put it.

If our diet and lifestyle are in the direction of positivity and purity, we rise up. If they're in the direction of negativity and cruelty, we don't move into the higher areas. When we drop the physical body, we will be at the same vibrational level we have attained up to that point. If we become established in the highest chakra, we live in the most refined level of the universe —pure light. Here are a few qualities of that level:

- We're young again. I mean, that would be a waste of getting to the highest level if we had to still be stiff, gray, vulnerable, crotchety old people. It doesn't happen like that. Just as first thing in the morning after a good sleep your face is relaxed and you feel good, so at the highest level you are youthful, relaxed, and feeling good.

- Do you need to breathe or worry about maybe having to stop breathing? No. You are light, and you are living in light. You don't need food, as you sometimes hear about certain highly evolved yogis. That worry is gone. You are scintillating energy all the time.

- You live in a translucent body. It's a body. But it's a body of light.

- When you want something, it just literally materializes right there. You don't need to ask. Your mental power is so strong that any thought is the first impulse of the universe. Cadillac? Don't need it. You can be anywhere with just the thought. Whatever you want you manifest. You can create anything just by thinking.

- How about companionship? Isn't it lonely being a light body? Your friends can't see you. Not to worry. Everybody is there. All the loved ones you have cared about. Your father and his father and his, your mother and her mother and hers. Everyone.

- How's your memory in a light body? Do you lose it? Actually you do, but not for the reason you think. It's not that your brain begins to lose its proper circuitry. It's the opposite. Your brain works perfectly. You don't need memory. Intuition is perfectly sharp. Anything you want to know, you know.

- What if you're on the path but still not quite there? If you haven't gained the light body, the rules of the game are quite straightforward. You have to come back to a human body and try again.

- How do you feel? You're in bliss most of the time. You're getting so much pleasure from the beauty and harmony everywhere. You're in ecstasy.

- In Vedic terms, you are only satisfied when prakriti (the body) is completely evolved and purusha (the silent pure consciousness) is fully expressed. When Shiva (silence) and Shakti (expressed level) are fully together, then you have everything.

What Do You Do When You're a Light Body?

Many people think that they're in no hurry to evolve to the highest levels because life will be boring at those high levels. It's actually the opposite. There's a lot going on, and a lot to do. If the body is completely purified, that span of time after the gross body drops off is quite as fulfilling and thrilling as the time with the physical body. Your senses are the super senses described in the chapter about powers. Death is no longer much of a concern, as you are at least as immortal as the universe itself and probably as the field of pure consciousness itself.

If you become a light body, you are immune to pain of all kinds. You are over-the-top, ecstatically fulfilled. You know everything. You can do everything. You can be anything. Anywhere in space and time. And now, thanks to epigenetics and DNA, that possibility of becoming a fulfilled light body emerges from the fog of human history.

The purpose of life is to perfect the genome. Epigenetics now affirms that we can do that. Switch on and off the right genes. Perfect yourself. Become a light body.

Summary and
Sweeping Implications

This Changes Everything. Let Us Count the Ways.

The implications of epigenetics hand-in-hand with Ayurvedic concepts stretch beyond the imagination. In a few short chapters, we have turned many current perceptions of health and life on their heads. Let's review the implications. Here's the Top 10 list:

10.
Ayurveda Takes the Lead in the Emerging Field of Epigenetics

In matters of health, we have for some generations been turning automatically to Western medicine. Ayurveda, when in the conversation at all, was one of a collection of alternative practices, along with homeopathy, acupuncture, traditional Chinese medicine, and a few other non-mainstream, loosely regulated, purely tangential health practices. Here we now have a focus on something that is highlighted in Western medicine—namely, DNA. What we have found, though, is that Ayurveda comes to the table armed with an understanding of the underside, or, more accurately, the *in*side of the material under consideration, of that newly valued and studied DNA.

Epigenetics has raised DNA from a somewhat manageable and predictable substance into a roiling mass of ever-changing, ever-widening expressions and emerging possibilities. Ayurveda has a long tradition, several millennia long, of working with the subjective side of life, and it has the systems for doing so. What Ayurveda has been doing correlates with what we call epigenetics today. No one expected such a thing to occur. Ayurveda is not just in the mix now. It is in the center of it all.

9.
Western Medicine Has to Become Aware of Ayurveda's Knowledge

A necessary corollary to the rise of Ayurveda in this context is the necessity for Western medicine to become aware of Ayurvedic knowledge and methodologies and to start incorporating them in their approach. Western medicine works with the physical body and treats disease. With sickness as prevalent as it is, we need this knowledge now more than ever. But when we enter the paradigm-shifting world of epigenetics, Western medicine is left at the gate. For starters, it should emphasize prevention, which is a primary consideration with epigenetics. And the saga is not over once a cell is free from disease. Epigenetics applies to healthy cells as well.

Second, Western medicine is not putting attention on the "other" side of DNA—consciousness and the energy fields, which are much more powerful than the grosser levels. Third, it does not address the profound aspect of bliss, or any of the higher possibilities we have discussed, such as healing abilities, enlightenment (or the gaining of the light body).

8.
Metaphysics Becomes Physical

Another transformation of our time is that metaphysics suddenly finds itself exposed as more or less untestable theoretical abstraction. Metaphysics has always been the primary domain for discussing spirituality because spirituality asks questions in the abstract. "Is there a spirit?" "Is there a God?" "How do we change the spirit?" "Which is more powerful, mind or body?" "Does mind really exist?" "Does body really exist?" Most spiritual seekers nestled comfortably into metaphysics by default. What did hard, scientific evidence have to offer them? Operating outside the physical realm preceded the current world, where all of a sudden the metaphysical is staring directly at us as something undeniably material— DNA. The metaphysical has become physical.

7.
Even Religion Becomes Physical

Religion has always been the domain of theological discussion and fully-worked-out abstract argument. It has also offered guidelines on lifestyle and behavior. For example, the Ten Commandments are do's and don'ts that comprise a set of standards for conduct. Now, we know that these standards are part of the physical field of epigenetics. Follow religion's advice, and your DNA leads you to health and happiness. Violate it, and your body protests with sickness and depression.

6.
Past Lives and Future Lives Enter the Conversation

Suggesting that we may have had past lives was previously cause for derision, or at least indifference. What did we really know about past lives, and where did we know it from? What evidence did we have? Did someone claim to have a memory of it? Did a soothsayer of some sort tell you about your previous life or lives? There was just nothing solid to hold on to. Now, though, it is found in our DNA. The legacy of our fathers and mothers and theirs and theirs shows up. And the legacy of our own behavior shows up. Some may still debate whether or not the DNA truly shows those previous lives, or predicts future ones, but we now know that we have somewhere concrete to look.

5.
Chakras Take Center Stage

Chakras were not really in the conversation in medicine. We couldn't touch them. We couldn't see them. We couldn't verify their effects. We thought of them as fascinating folklore, not solid enough to be a real consideration for treating health. Now, with energy systems and consciousness seen as the keys to a healthy epigenetic feedback loop, these traditional energy distributors are central players. They distribute the life force, kundalini. What are they and how do they behave? How can we get them working properly for health and more? They're not forgotten any longer.

4.
Karma Becomes Physical

When the forward-looking generation of the 1960s in the Western world began to speak of "karma," everyone got a good chuckle. "Bad karma" was the most common phrase, and it referred to something happening, like tripping over a log, or getting turned down for a job, or losing a boyfriend or girlfriend. People knew it had something to do with things happening, *but that was it.* It certainly was not scientific. It certainly did not have to do with the inner workings of our own bodies. It was not measurable. It was not central to our path of life on the earth. It was a joke, mostly, and a term that only the hip and current knew. Now it can be considered to have risen up as the central principle of all action. If karma is physical and tracked by the DNA, though, it may seem to merit a second look from its many doubters. Karma is not tracked off in the sky but rather in the body itself.

Now we know that whatever we do or think or don't do or don't think gets registered in a supernormal recording system, our DNA. We know that the old idea of "what you do comes back to you" is now the epigenetic feedback loop. Karma can now be seen to be a description of how life is operating, and the central rule for how to live, evolve, and rise above sickness to a higher life.

3.
Kundalini Comes Out of Obscurity

If the rise of chakras is dramatic in how we look at life, the rise of kundalini is absolutely, earthshakingly transforming to how we regard our life. Kundalini, that old, unknown, misunderstood snake at the base of the spine, is now the life force in the body, and the mechanism for waking up the DNA in every nucleated cell of the body. Everyone who thought about it at all, thought of it as contained along the spine. Now we're discovering that what we have known as kundalini is everywhere, just as cells are everywhere, and it causes the brain of the cells, the DNA, to function. No kundalini, no life. Powerful kundalini, powerful life.

2.
New Age Comes of Age

Who were the custodians of "chakras" and "kundalini" and "karma" and "consciousness" and "auras" and all the terms and sub-terms that go along with them? The "New Agers." And New Agers were felt by the masses of mankind to be wishful thinkers, a bit soft, talking among themselves to little or no purpose. Their numbers may have been legion, but many of the participants were more tourists than participants. You could fade in and out of New Age, and nobody much noticed or minded.

Now, what we call the New Agers are sitting on top of the central knowledge of the nervous system and its innermost functioning. It doesn't mean they're vindicated or their ideas and beliefs have been verified, but it means that both this vindication and verification are now good possibilities. Credibility is coming from Western medicine researchers in their function as the tester and validator for all those terms that New Agers have been passing back and forth so glibly. Side players until now, New Agers suddenly sit right at the head of the table. Their time has come, and Western medicine has brought it to them.

1.
The Goal of Life Becomes Physical

All the rest of the transformations that epigenetics brings to us pale beside a single one, which is that the goal of life is now physical.

Instead of debating about the goal of life or essentially ignoring the question, we can look at it squarely and say unequivocally that the goal of life is to get the DNA working properly, and epigenetics is the way to do it.

To be blunt about it, the goal of life is to be equal to death and, indeed, unaffected by it. Death is all around us every day. Just as life springs up continuously, death is also continuous. Plants, animals, the day, and the season all rise up in life and continue onto death. Everyone knows that death is part of life, but most people feel that the best thing is not to think too much about it because you can't do anything about it anyway.

Now you can. Be systematic about getting your lifestyle, diet, environment and ways to handle stress working for you, and use whatever tools work best for bringing kundalini zinging through the cells. Do it well enough, and the wonders you have heard about with yogis and extraordinary people from the past can be yours. The goal is to head in that direction.

There are many resting stations along the way where the idea of death becomes more and more tolerable and bliss becomes more and more the style of your existence. And there, when you get it all completely right, is the light body. You are light at your basis. We know how to get that light flowing more and more through our cells. We do it with the epigenetic feedback loop.

The purpose of life is to perfect the genome. Epigenetics affirms that we can now do that. You can switch on and off the right genes. Perfect yourself. Become a light body. We know what to do to get there, and is it ever worth doing.

Glossary

Ayurveda – (also called Ayurvedic Medicine) from the Sanskrit words *ayus*, meaning "life" and *veda*, meaning "science" or "knowledge," literally means the complete knowledge of the totality of life. It is the knowledge of how to bring individual and collective life into accord with the laws of nature that govern life. It not only adds years to one's life, it also adds life to one's years. The motto of Ayurveda is "Ayurvedo Amritanam," meaning Ayurveda is for those who desire immortality. Ayurveda began in the ancient Vedic times of India over 5,000 years ago. Indians today use Ayurvedic medicine either exclusively or combined with conventional Western medicine. It is also practiced in various forms in Southeast Asia. Ayurveda was introduced to the United States during the New Age movement in the late 1960s and 1970s and became more popular with the general public during the 1980s and 1990s. Ayurveda has been introduced in European countries, Australia, New Zealand, Russia, South America, Canada, Africa and other countries.

Ayurveda is strongly prevention-oriented and provides a variety of treatments for chronic disorders and maintenance of good health. Different modalities which Ayurveda uses include herbal, mineral, and other compounds, and specialized preparations called rasayanas. Other recommendations include diet, lifestyle, daily and seasonal routine, meditation, breathing exercises, yoga asanas, daily massage, environmental recommendations, and panchakarma, a physiological purification technique. Key concepts include a system of interconnectivity of people among each other and the universe and a belief of the connection of the body's constitution with universal life forces.

Chakras – The seven distribution centers of prana (energy) in the area of the spine and brain that enliven the physical and subtle bodies. These centers of concentrated energy radiate energy in the physiology through channels known as nadis. Chakras correlate with the endocrine glands and nerve plexuses.

DNA – Deoxyribonucleic acid. DNA is comprised of multiple nucleotides which are composed of nitrogenous bases added to a sugar and a phosphate group. DNA is present in all the nucleated cells of the body. A gene is a segment of DNA that can be transcribed or replicated. The totality of all the genes in the physiology forms the genome.

Epigenetics – Refers to external modification to DNA that turns genes on and off, affecting gene expression, which can have transgenerational effects and/or inherited expression states. This occurs without changes in the DNA sequence. This process produces a change in the phenotype without a change in the genotype.

Genome – The totality of all the genes in the physiology forms the genome.

Genotype – Refers to the part of the genetic makeup that determines specific characteristics of an individual. It is responsible for the development of the phenotype of the individual.

Kundalini – Individualized life force that rises in the central channel in the spinal area, opening up the chakras to reach the top chakra, to merge with Purusha or Consciousness. Kundalini also functions in the DNA for its expression.

Marma – The marma points are deep-seated, vitally important physio-anatomical structures that reflect prana or life force on the surface of the body. Marmas connect to the chakras and nadis. There are 108 marma points on the physical body.

Nadis – Channels that emanate from the chakras, through which prana flows to the different parts of the body to sustain life.

Panchakarma – Ayurvedic purification therapy, which removes impurities from the shrotas, the physiological channels in the body.

Phenotype – Refers to the physical properties of an individual—appearance, development, and behavior. The phenotype is determined by the genotype, as well as environmental influences as it develops and inherited epigenetic factors.

Prakriti – This term can have different meanings. It refers to power (shakti), female, psychophysiological constitution or body type in Ayurveda. The meaning depends on the context in which it is used.

Prana – It is said to be an impulse of abstract absolute Being. Being is the absolute existence of unmanifested nature. Vibration of Being to manifest is referred to as prana. This is the life principle of the physical world. There are two kinds of Prana: cosmic vibratory energy in the universe, and Prana in the human body that sustains life.

RNA – Ribonucleic acid. RNA is transcribed from DNA and translated to form proteins. Messenger RNA (mRNA) carries the transcribed information. Transfer RNA (tRNA) translates the information and transfers the amino acids required for the formation of proteins.

Shrotas – Refers to different types of channels in the physiology through which material flows, e.g. blood vessels, gastrointestinal tract, etc.

Endnotes

1. www.go.osu.edu/fuzzyhologram

2. Champagne, F.A., Rissman, E.F. "Behavioral Epigenetics: A New Frontier in the Study of Hormones and Behavior." *Hormones and Behavior* 2011;59(3):277-278.

3. Champagne, F.A., Mashoodh, R. "Genes in Context: Gene-Environment Interplay and the Origins of Individual Differences in Behavior." *Current Directions in Psychological Science* 2009;18(3):127-131.

4. Lester, B.M., Tronick, E., Nestler, E., et al. "Behavioral Epigenetics." *Annals of the New York Academy of Sciences* 2011;1226:14-33.

5. Lewkowicz, D.J. "The Biological Implausibility of the Nature-Nurture Dichotomy and What it Means for the Study of Infancy." *Infancy* 2011;16(4):331-367.

6. Paul, A.M. *Origins: How the Nine Months Before Birth Shape the Rest of Our Lives* (New York: Free Press, 2010).

7. Powledge, T.M. "Behavioral Epigenetics: How Nurture Shapes Nature." *BioScience* 2011;61(8):588-592.

8. Alegria-Torres, J.A., Baccarelli, A., Bollati, V. "Epigenetics and Lifestyle." *Epigenomics* 2011;3(3):267-277.

9. Haluskova, J. "Epigenetic Studies in Human Diseases." *Folia Biologica (Praha)* 2010;56(3):83–96.

10. Dopico, X.C., Evangelou, M., Ferreira, R.C., et al. "Widespread Seasonal Gene Expression Reveals Annual Differences in Human Immunity and Physiology." *Nature Communications* 2015:6:7000. doi: 10.1038/ncomms8000

11. Skinner, M.K. "Environmental Stress and Epigenetic Transgenerational Inheritance." *BMC Medicine* 2014;12:153. doi: 10.1186/s12916-014-0153-y.

12. Ornish, D., Magbanua, M.J.M., Weidner, G., et al. "Changes in Prostate Gene Expression in Men Undergoing an Intensive Nutrition and Lifestyle Intervention." *Proceedings of the National Academy of Sciences USA* 2008;105(24):8369-8374.

13. Fagan, J. "Consciousness-Based Health Care: Modulating Gene Expression to Achieve System-Wide Balance and Integration Through the Ayurvedic Modality, Transcendental Meditation." Presented at the International Ayurveda Congress, London, April 1-3, 2017.

14. Sharma, H., Mishra, R.K., Meade, J.G. *The Answer to Cancer* (New York: SelectBooks, 2002).

15. Schneider, R.H., Grim, C.E., Rainforth, M.V., et al. "Stress Reduction in the Secondary Prevention of Cardiovascular Disease. Randomized, Controlled Trial of Transcendental Meditation and Health Education in Blacks." *Circulation: Cardiovascular Quality and Outcomes* 2012;5:750-758.

16. Frawley, D., Ranade, S., Lele, A. *Ayurveda and Marma Therapy* (Twin Lakes, WI: Lotus Press, 2003).

17. Hunt, V. "Electronic Evidence of Auras, Chakras in UCLA Study." *Brain/ Mind Bulletin* 1978;3(9):1-2.

18. Miller, R. "Bridging the Gap: An Interview with Valerie Hunt, Ed. D." *Science of Mind*, 1983, p. 12.

19. http://gdvcamera.com

20. Braden, G. *Awakening to Zero Point* (Bellevue, WA: Radio Bookstore Press, 1997).

21. Narayanan, C.R. personal communication, 2015.

22. Joshi, S.K. *Marma Science and Principles of Marma Therapy* (Delhi: Vani Publications, March 2014).

23. Singh, R.H., Singh, N.B., Udupa, K.N. "A Study of Tridosha as Neurohumors." *Journal of Research in Ayurveda and Siddha* 1980;1(1):1-20.

24. Prasher, B., Negi, S., Aggarwal, S., et al. "Whole Genome Expression and Biochemical Correlates of Extreme Constitutional Types Defined in Ayurveda." *Journal of Translational Medicine* 2008;6:48. doi: 10.1186/1479-5876-6-48

25. Patwardhan, B., Joshi, K., Chopra, A. "Classification of Human Population Based on HLA Gene Polymorphism and the Concept of Prakriti in Ayurveda." *Journal of Alternative and Complementary Medicine* 2005;11(2): 349-353.

26. Dey, S., Pahwa, P. "Prakriti and Its Associations with Metabolism, Chronic Diseases, and Genotypes: Possibilities of Newborn Screening and a Lifetime of Personalized Prevention." *Journal of Ayurveda and Integrative Medicine* 2014;5(1):15-24.

27. Mahalle, N.P., Kulkarni, M.V., Pendse, N.M., et al. "Association of Constitutional Type of Ayurveda with Cardiovascular Risk Factors, Inflammatory Markers and Insulin Resistance." *Journal of Ayurveda and Integrative Medicine* 2012;3(3):150-157.

28. Tiwari, S., Gehlot, S., Tiwari, S.K., et al. "Effect of Walking (Aerobic Isotonic Exercise) on Physiological Variants with Special Reference to Prameha (Diabetes Mellitus) as per Prakriti." *AYU* 2012;33(1):44-49.

29. Bhalerao, S., Deshpande, T., Thatte, U. "Prakriti (Ayurvedic Concept of Constitution) and Variations in Platelet Aggregation." *BMC Complementary and Alternative Medicine* 2012;12:248. doi: 10.1186/1472-6882-12-248

30. Aggarwal, S., Negi, S., Jha, P., et al. "EGLN1 Involvement in High-Altitude Adaptation Revealed Through Genetic Analysis of Extreme Constitution Types Defined in Ayurveda." *Proceedings of the National Academy of Sciences USA* 2010;107(44):18961-18966.

31. Manyam, B.V., Kumar, A. "Ayurvedic Constitution (Prakruti) Identifies Risk Factor of Developing Parkinson's Disease." *Journal of Alternative and Complementary Medicine* 2013;19(7):644-649.

32. Ghodke, Y., Joshi, K., Patwardhan, B. "Traditional Medicine to Modern Pharmacogenomics: Ayurveda Prakriti Type and CYP2C19 Gene Polymorphism Associated with Metabolic Variability." *Evid Based Complementary Alternative Medicine* 2011;2011:249528. doi: 10.1093/ecam/nep206.

33. Hagelin, J. "Maharishi Vedic Medicine is Ultra-Modern, Cutting-Edge Medicine – Unified Field Based Medicine." Presented at the International Ayurveda Congress, London, April 1-3, 2017.

34. Hagelin, J.S. "Is Consciousness the Unified Field? A Field Theorist's Perspective." *Modern Science and Vedic Science* 1987;1(1):29-87.

35. Grace, D.M. *Beyond Bodies: Gender, Literature and the Enigma of Consciousness* (Amsterdam, The Netherlands: Brill Rodopi, 2014).

36. Sharma, H., Clark, C. *Ayurvedic Healing* (London: Singing Dragon, 2012), pp. 192–194.

37. Taube, J.S. "Head Direction Cells Recorded in the Anterior Thalamic Nuclei of Freely Moving Rats." *Journal of Neuroscience* 1995;15(1):70-86.

38. Rajeswari, K.R., Satyanarayana, M., Sanker, P.V., et al. "Effect of Extremely Low Frequency Magnetic Field on Serum Cholinesterase in Humans and Animals." *Indian Journal of Experimental Biology* 1985;23:194-197.

39. Singh, T.C.N., Gnanam, A. "Studies on the Effect of Sound Waves of Nadeshwaram on the Growth and Yield of Paddy." *Journal of Annamalai University* 1965;16:78-99.

40. Hicks, C.B. "Growing Corn to Music." *Popular Mechanics* 1963;119:118-121,183.

41. Retallack, D. *The Sound of Music and Plants.* (Marina del Ray, CA: Devorss and Co., 1973), pp. 20-33.

42. Sharma, H., Kauffman, E., Stephens, R. "Effect of Sama Veda and Hard Rock Music on Growth of Human Cancer Cell Lines in Vitro." *AYU* 2008;29(1):1-8.

43. Mishra, L.C. (ed). *Scientific Basis for Ayurvedic Therapies* (New York: CRC Press, 2004).

44. Puri, H.S. *Rasayana: Ayurvedic Herbs for Longevity and Rejuvenation* (London: Taylor and Francis, 2003).

45. Ornish, D., Lin, J., Chan, J.M., et al. "Effect of Comprehensive Lifestyle Changes on Telomerase Activity and Telomere Length in Men with Biopsy-Proven Low-Risk Prostate Cancer: 5-year Follow-up of a Descriptive Pilot Study." *Lancet Oncol* 2013;14:1112-1120.

46. Epel, E.S., Blackburn, E.H., Lin, J., et al. "Accelerated Telomere Shortening in Response to Life Stress." *Proceedings of the National Academy of Sciences USA* 2004;101(49):17312-17315.

47. Blackburn, E., Epel, E. *The Telomere Effect.* New York: Grand Central Publishing, 2017.

48. Jacobs, T.L., Epel, E.S., Lin, J., et al. "Intensive Meditation Training, Immune Cell Telomerase Activity, and Psychological Mediators." *Psychoneuroendocrinology* 2011;36:664-681.

49. Choi, J., Fauce, S.R., Effros, R.B. "Reduced Telomerase Activity in Human T Lymphocytes Exposed to Cortisol." *Brain, Behavior, and Immunity* 2008;22:600-605.

50. Sharma, H. "Meditation: Process and Effects." *AYU* 2015;36:233-237.

51. Arias, A.J., Steinberg, K., Banga, A., et al. "Systematic Review of the Efficacy of Meditation Techniques as Treatments for Medical Illness." *Journal of Alternative and Complementary Medicine* 2006;12(8):817-832.

52. Sharma, H.M. "Contemporary Ayurveda." In: Micozzi, M.S., ed. *Fundamentals of Complementary and Alternative Medicine. 4th edition.* St. Louis: Saunders Elsevier, 2011, pp. 495–508.

53. Sharma, H. "Integrating Ayurveda into Clinical Practice." In: Bhandari, C.M., Kulmatycki, L., eds. *Joga & Ajurweda W Badaniach Naukowych [Yoga and Ayurveda in Scientific Research].* Warsaw, Poland: BJ Sp. z o. o., 2014:45-64.

54. Gupta, S.C., Sung, B., Kim, J.H., et al. "Multitargeting by Turmeric, the Golden Spice: From Kitchen to Clinic." *Molecular Nutrition and Food Research* 2013;57:1510-1528.

55. Vayalil, P.K., Kuttan, G., Kuttan, R. "Protective Effects of Rasayanas on Cyclophosphamide- and Radiation-induced Damage." *Journal of Alternative and Complementary Medicine* 2002;8(6):787-796.

56. Govindarajan, R., Vijayakumar, M., Pushpangadan, P. "Antioxidant Approach to Disease Management and the Role of 'Rasayana' Herbs of Ayurveda." *J Ethnopharmacol* 2005;99:165-178.

57. Sharma, H., Chandola, H.M., Singh, G., et al. "Utilization of Ayurveda in Health Care: An Approach for Prevention, Health Promotion, and Treatment of Disease. Part 1 – Ayurveda, the Science of Life." *Journal of Alternative and Complementary Medicine* 2007;13(9):1011-1019.

58. Sharma, H., Chandola, H.M., Singh, G., et al. "Utilization of Ayurveda in Health Care: An Approach for Prevention, Health Promotion, and Treatment of Disease. Part 2 – Ayurveda in Primary Health Care." *Journal of Alternative and Complementary Medicine* 2007;13(10):1135-1150.

59. Sharma, H.M., Alexander, C.N. "Maharishi Ayurveda: Research Review. Part 2: Maharishi Ayurveda Herbal Food Supplements and Additional Strategies." *Complementary Medicine International* 1996;3(2):17-28.

60. Aggarwal, B.B., Yuan, W., Li, S., et al. "Curcumin-Free Turmeric Exhibits Anti-Inflammatory and Anticancer Activities: Identification of Novel Components of Turmeric." *Molecular Nutrition & Food Research* 2013;57:1529-1542.

61. Anand, P., Kunnumakkara, A.B., Newman, R.A., et al. "Bioavailability of Curcumin: Problems and Promises." *Molecular Pharmaceutics* 2007;4(6):807-818.

62. Hafner, M., Stepanek, M., Taylor, J., et al. "Why Sleep Matters—the Economic Costs of Insufficient Sleep: A Cross-Country Comparative Analysis." Santa Monica, CA: RAND Corporation, 2016. https://www.rand.org/pubs/research_reports/RR1791.html

63. Travis, F., Shear, J. "Focused Attention, Open Monitoring and Automatic Self-Transcending: Categories to Organize Meditations from Vedic, Buddhist and Chinese Traditions." *Consciousness and Cognition* 2010;19:1110-1118.

64. Travis, F., Arenander, A. "Cross-Sectional and Longitudinal Study of Effects of Transcendental Meditation Practice on Interhemispheric Frontal Asymmetry and Frontal Coherence." *International Journal of Neuroscience* 2006;116(12):1519-1538.

65. Streeter, C.C., Gerbarg, P.L., Saper, R.B., et al. "Effects of Yoga on the Autonomic Nervous System, Gamma-Aminobutyric Acid, and Allostasis in Epilepsy, Depression, and Post-Traumatic Stress Disorder." *Medical Hypotheses* 2012;78(5):571-579.

66. http://ejmas.com/pt/ptart_shin_0400.htm

67. O'Connell, D.F., Alexander, C.N., eds. *Self-Recovery: Treating Addictions Using Transcendental Meditation and Maharishi Ayur-Veda.* (New York: The Haworth Press, 1994).

68. Lutz, A., Greischar, L.L., Rawlings, N.B., et al. "Long-Term Meditators Self-Induce High-Amplitude Gamma Synchrony during Mental Practice." *Proceedings of the National Academy of Sciences USA* 2004;101(46):16369-16373.

69. Lazar, S.W., Kerr, C.E., Wasserman, R.H., et al. "Meditation Experience is Associated with Increased Cortical Thickness." *NeuroReport* 2005;16(17):1893-1897.

70. Jevning, R., Wallace, R.K., Beidebach, M. "The Physiology of Meditation: A Review. A Wakeful Hypometabolic Integrated Response." *Neuroscience and Biobehavioral Reviews* 1992;16:415-424.

71. Jevning, R., Wilson, A.F., Davidson, J.M. "Adrenocortical Activity during Meditation." *Hormones and Behavior* 1978;10(1):54-60.

72. Glaser, J.L., Brind, J.L., Vogelman, J.H., et al. "Elevated Serum Dehydroepiandrosterone Sulfate Levels in Practitioners of the Transcendental Meditation (TM) & TM-Sidhi Programs." *Journal of Behavioral Medicine* 1992;15(4):327-341.

73. Wallace, R.K., Dillbeck, M., Jacobe, E., et al. "The Effects of the Transcendental Meditation and TM-Sidhi Program on the Aging Process." *International Journal of Neuroscience* 1982;16(1):53-58.

74. Orme-Johnson, D. "Medical Care Utilization and the Transcendental Meditation Program." *Psychosomatic Medicine* 1987;49(5):493-507.

75. Barnes, V.A., Orme-Johnson, D.W. "Clinical and Pre-Clinical Applications of the Transcendental Meditation Program in the Prevention and Treatment of Essential Hypertension and Cardiovascular Disease in Youth and Adults." *Current Hypertension Reviews* 2006;2(3):207-218.

76. Herron, R.E. "Changes in Physician Costs among High-Cost Transcendental Meditation Practitioners Compared with High-Cost Nonpractitioners over 5 Years." *American Journal of Health Promotion* 2011;26(1):56-60.

77. Chan, D., Woollacott, M. "Effects of Level of Meditation Experience on Attentional Focus: Is the Efficiency of Executive or Orientation Networks Improved?" *Journal of Alternative and Complementary Medicine* 2007;13(6):651-657.

78. Alexander, E. *Proof of Heaven: A Neurosurgeon's Journey into the Afterlife* (New York: Simon & Schuster, 2012).

79. Bolte Taylor, J. *My Stroke of Insight: A Brain Scientist's Personal Journey* (New York: Penguin, 2008).

80. Stevenson, I. *Twenty Cases Suggestive of Reincarnation* (Charlottesville, VA: University of Virginia Press, 1980).

81. Atwater, P.M.H. *Near-Death Experiences: The Rest of the Story* (Charlottesville, VA: Hampton Roads Publishing Co., 2011).

82. Burpo, T., Vincent, L. *Heaven Is for Real: A Little Boy's Astounding Story of His Trip to Heaven and Back* (Nashville, TN: Thomas Nelson, 2010).

83. Carter, C. *Science and the Afterlife Experience: Evidence for the Immortality of Consciousness* (Rochester, VT: Inner Traditions, 2012).

84. Eadie, B.J. *Embraced by the Light* (Placerville, CA: Gold Leaf Press, 1992).

85. Holden, J.M., Greyson, B., James, D., eds. *The Handbook of Near-Death Experiences: Thirty Years of Investigation* (Santa Barbara, CA: Praeger, 2009).

86. Kübler-Ross, E. *On Life After Death* (Berkeley, CA: Ten Speed Press, 1991).

87. Moody, R.A. *Life After Life: The Investigation of a Phenomenon—Survival of Bodily Death* (New York: HarperCollins, 2001).

88. Moody, R., Perry, P. *Glimpses of Eternity: Sharing a Loved One's Passage from This Life to the Next* (New York: Guideposts, 2010).

89. Moorjani, A. *Dying to Be Me: My Journey from Cancer, to Near Death, to True Healing* (Carlsbad, CA: Hay House, 2012).

90. Piper, D., Murphey, C. *90 Minutes in Heaven: A True Story of Death and Life* (Grand Rapids, MI: Revell, 2004).

91. Stevenson, I. *Children Who Remember Previous Lives: A Question of Reincarnation* (Jefferson, NC: McFarland, 2001).

92. Tompkins, P. *The Modern Book of the Dead: A Revolutionary Perspective on Death, the Soul, and What Really Happens in the Life to Come* (New York: Atria Books, 2012).

93. Tucker, J.B. *Life Before Life: A Scientific Investigation of Children's Memories of Previous Lives* (New York: St. Martin's, 2005).

94. Kessler, R. *The Sins of the Father: Joseph P. Kennedy and the Dynasty He Founded* (New York: Grand Central Publishing, 1996).

95. Flint, M.S., Baum, A., Chambers, W.H., et al. "Induction of DNA Damage, Alteration of DNA Repair and Transcriptional Activation by Stress Hormones." *Psychoneuroendocrinology* 2007;32(5):470-479.

96. Hara, M.R., Kovacs, J.J., Whalen, E.J., et al. "A Stress Response Pathway Regulates DNA Damage through B2-Adrenoreceptors and B-Arrestin-1." *Nature* 2011;477(7364):349-353.

97. Hara, M.R., Sachs, B.D., Caron, M.G., et al. "Pharmacological Blockade of a B2ar-B-Arrestin-1 Signaling Cascade Prevents the Accumulation of DNA Damage in a Behavioral Stress Model. *Cell Cycle* 2013;12(2):219-224.

98. http://www.bibliotecapleyades.net/ciencia/ciencia_genetica04.htm.

99. Motz, J. "Everyone an Energy Healer." The Treat V Conference, Santa Fe, NM. *Advances: The Journal of Mind-Body Health* 1993;9.

100. Rein, G., McCraty, R. "Structural Changes in Water and DNA Associated with New Physiologically Measurable States." *Journal of Scientific Exploration* 1994;8(3):438-439.

101. Lancer, D. "The Healing Power of Eros." *International Journal of Emergency Mental Health* 2015;17(1):213-218.

102. Wallace, R.K. *The Physiology of Consciousness* (Fairfield, IA: Maharishi International University Press, 1993).

Index

About the Authors

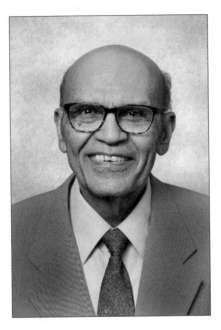

Hari Sharma, MD, DABIHM, FACN, DABP, FCAP, FRCPC

Hari Sharma, MD, a Western physician with an impressive list of titles, is in reality a game changer. A reality changer. For instance, his book on cancer is not simply "Cancer Prevention"; it is *The Answer to Cancer*. That is, he is looking to revolutionize and reform the approach to cancer as a whole, not just chip away at it. His other book on disease is not just "Some Effective Approaches to a Tough Problem." It is *Freedom from Disease*.

Dr. Sharma's career represents a synthesis of the modern-day knowledge of Western medicine and the ancient knowledge of the natural, comprehensive Vedic system of health care. He has extensively studied, practiced, and researched both systems. In addition, Dr. Sharma has studied under many spiritual teachers and has extensive knowledge of the

Vedas and various spiritual practices. He had the honor of being named Fellow of the National Academy of Ayurveda by the Ministry of Health and Family Welfare, Government of India.

Dr. Sharma is Professor Emeritus and former Director of the Division of Cancer Prevention and Natural Products Research in the Department of Pathology, College of Medicine, at The Ohio State University in Columbus, Ohio.* He is a diplomate of the American Board of Integrative Holistic Medicine and the American Board of Pathology, a Fellow of the American College of Nutrition and Emeritus Fellow of the Royal College of Physicians and Surgeons of Canada, and a member of various national and international professional societies. Dr. Sharma is past Chair of the Integrated Medicine Committee of National AAPI (American Association of Physicians of Indian Origin). He has been practicing Ayurveda at The Ohio State University Integrative Medicine clinic since its inception in 2005.*

Dr. Sharma is a frequent lecturer at conferences worldwide. He has published over 150 research articles and authored/coauthored five books related to Ayurveda, including *Ayurvedic Healing* and *Awakening Nature's Healing Intelligence*.

*Institutional endorsement not implied.

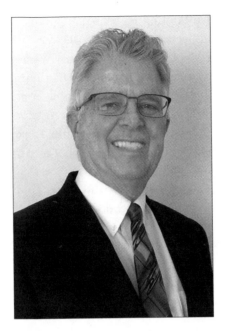

James G. Meade, PhD

Writer James G. Meade, PhD, is a veteran of numerous skirmishes to transform human life on earth, including the rise of software as our everyday reality and, on the consciousness front, the practice of meditation and related complementary-medicine technologies. He championed several emerging technologies for companies like Microsoft and IBM and was one of the first authors in the ground-breaking Dummies series (which brought right-brained thinking into left-brained computer and business writing).

Meade collaborated with Dr. Sharma on *The Answer to Cancer*, which became a word-of-mouth sensation passed hand to hand by those who have read it. "It makes all that technical material digestible, even fun," readers have said, often devouring the 220-page book in one sitting.

A literary man with a technical bent, Meade has published thirty previous books and sold more than 750,000 copies around the world. His *The Human Resources Software Handbook*, published with leading business publisher John Wiley Publishing, helped companies ease from tracking employees on spreadsheets to doing so on the web with multipurpose software. He has published five titles in the For Dummies series, one of the best known and most successful book series of all time.

But resolving the human condition has been his quest, and he has taught meditation to thousands of people across the United States and in Hong Kong, Nepal, Jamaica, Hungary, and Tanzania. A sought-after speaker, he just completed a tour in Asia that took him to Hong Kong, Viet Nam, Cambodia, and Thailand.

His PhD is in English, from Northwestern University "with distinguished commendation." He attended graduate school on an NDEA Fellowship. A journalist at heart, he has been a columnist for several publications, including "Information Week."